Juice, Blend, Taste

by

THE
⊗
JUICERY

EXPERT GOODNESS

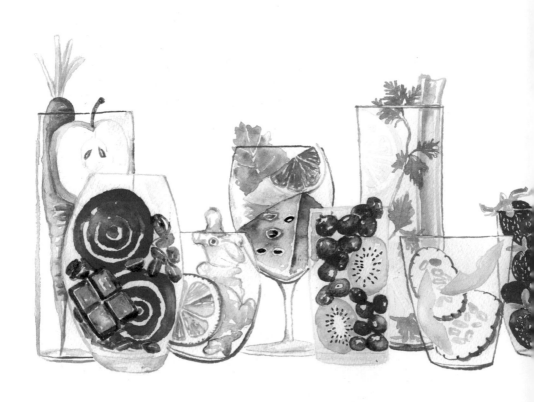

JUICE

fruits, vegetables, herbs & spices

BLEND

nut milks, coconut water, yogurt & superfoods

TASTE

fresh juices, sweet & savory smoothies, booster shots,
sparkling drinks, iced teas & warm infusions that taste as
good as they are good for you from the experts at

THE ⊗ JUICERY

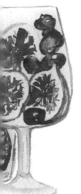

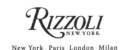

RIZZOLI NEW YORK

New York · Paris · London · Milan

First published in the United States of America in 2014
by Rizzoli International Publications, Inc.
300 Park Avenue South
New York, NY 10010
www.rizzoliusa.com

Design by Claudia Wu
Edited by Martynka Wawrzyniak

2014 2015 2016 2017 / 10 9 8 7 6 5 4 3 2 1

Distributed in the U.S. trade by Random House, New York

Printed in China

ISBN: 978-0-7893-2746-8

Library of Congress Control Number: 2014931974

This book would not have been possible without the love and support of many.

To my parents, my brother, Anu, and Neal for their never-ending support and love; the incredible Rizzoli team of Charles Miers, Nicky Clendening, and Martynka Wawrzyniak; Liana Krissoff, Katrine van Wyk, Jesse Kanelos Weiner, Marie Soh, and Claudia Wu for bringing it to life; Jason Harler and Tanya Hughes for their boundless creative energy; all of the amazing visionaries who contributed their time and delicious recipes to this book and who are an everyday source of inspiration; Georgia Fendley and the whole Construct team for their creative vision; the Equinox team for giving me a start; Bernie Gallagher, Garreth Walsh, Patrick King, and the whole team at the Doyle Collection for being the very best of partners; Des McDonald for his generosity of spirit and sage advice; Frank Lipman, Joe Cross, Dhrumil Purohit, Renae Kerber, and Reema Shroff for their support and encouragement; and Alejandro Junger for my first juice and starting me on this journey. —Cindy Palusamy

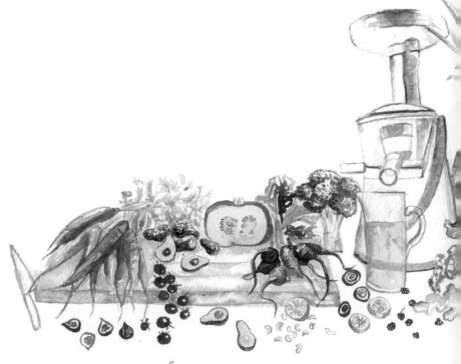

CONTENTS

· · · · · · · · · · ·

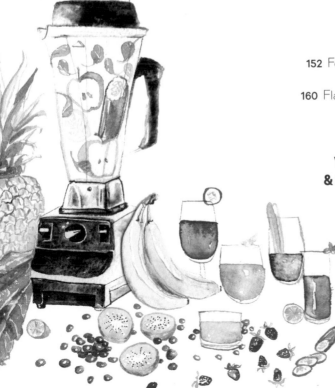

INTRODUCTION

The Juicery brings to life modern-day healthy living from the top global names in health, nutrition, and beauty. Launched in London in 2012, we teamed up with the brightest lights in the fields of nutrition and integrative medicine for some "expert goodness" to answer all your daily healthy-food needs. We believe that the sheer pleasure of experiencing great juice and food should lead the march toward a healthier, happier life. Gone are the days of the crunchy "this *must* be good for me!" approach to health food. Our focus is on recipes that taste as good as they are for you.

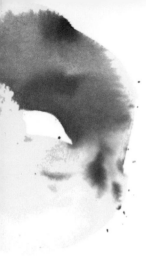

JUICING AND BLENDING 101

EQUIPMENT

Whether you're juicing or blending—or both—there are only a few pieces of kitchen equipment you'll need for the recipes in this book. Start with a sturdy cutting board and a good sharp knife or two, a vegetable peeler you're comfortable with (ones with a Y-shape seem to work best for most people), and a natural-bristle brush for scrubbing produce. A salad spinner or a large colander or sieve will be useful for rinsing bunches of greens and herbs.

What you'll need for juicing: You can make fruit and vegetable juices with nothing more than a high-speed blender and a couple layers of rinsed and squeezed cheesecloth or a nut-milk bag for straining out the solids. This is, as you can imagine, not a fuss-free process. If you're going to make juices on a regular basis—say, once a week or more—you'll probably want to invest in a good-quality juicer to do the job efficiently. There are many, many juicers on the market, in all sizes and price ranges. Most of them fall into one of two categories: centrifugal juicers and mastication or cold-press juicers. Centrifugal juicers, which work by shredding or grinding the produce and spinning the resulting pulp at high speed to extract the juice, are less expensive than mastication juicers and might be a good option if you're just starting to juice and are looking for an affordable entry-level machine, but there are some drawbacks. First, some centrifugal juicers can't extract as much juice from fruits and vegetables, which means you'll need to feed more produce into it for each glass of juice. Second, some argue that the centrifugal process generates heat and oxygen, which may damage enzymes and nutrients in the produce. There is no clear evidence of significant degradation, but you will notice a more immediate oxidation process. If you're using a centrifugal juicer, it's best to drink your juice immediately after you make it.

The higher-end mastication juicers, on the other hand, work by a technique similar to that of a mortar and pestle (or your teeth), grinding the fruits and vegetables and then squeezing out the juice. The process takes a little longer (these juicers are sometimes referred to as "slow juicers"), but it also yields more juice, and because no heat is generated and oxygen production is kept to a minimum, the resulting juice retains more of the whole foods' nutritive value and can be kept a bit longer than juice made with a centrifugal juicer. A mastication juicer is a bigger investment up front, but the increased yields can make up the difference fairly quickly.

One thing to keep in mind when you're shopping for a juicer is cleanup. Whatever kind of juicer you choose, after every use you'll need to take it apart and rinse it thoroughly. So the fewer parts (and crevices and seams in those parts) a juicer has, the easier it will be to clean—and the more likely you'll be to use it frequently.

What you'll need for blending: There are even more blenders on the market than there are juicers, in an even wider price range (think: paper bag versus Birkin bag). Most standard kitchen blenders will do just fine with your average smoothie of berries, bananas, avocados, even tender spinach. But if you plan to include a lot of dark leafy greens like kale or collards, hard raw produce like apples or beets, frozen fruits or vegetables, or ice, a more powerful high-speed blender is the way to go. The gold standard in blenders is Vitamix, used by many top chefs and at many juice and smoothie bars. Vitamix and other high-speed blenders can reduce virtually any ingredient to a smooth, creamy consistency for perfectly chunk-free soups and smoothies. Despite their powerful motors, they are surprisingly gentle on your produce and don't get hot enough to destroy enzymes or nutrients. High-speed blenders are also great for making homemade nut milks and nut butters.

You might also consider a small portable blender, often called a "bullet," for carrying along when you travel so you can take full advantage of good-quality local produce and maintain your commitment to healthful, delicious meals and pick-me-ups wherever you are. They make a single serving at a time in a cup that's turned upside down over the blades.

What you'll need for making iced teas, warm infusions, and sparkling drinks: A small saucepan or a teakettle along with a heatproof bowl for heating water and infusing it with herbs are the basics. In some cases a blender and a fine-mesh sieve for straining are required as well. Have a good supply of ice cubes, made with filtered water, on hand.

GETTING READY

Juicing and blending don't require much in the way of preparation, and you'll notice as you flip through this book that the recipes are all eminently simple and straightforward. That said, some ingredients will need a turn under cold running water, a knife, and/or a peeler before you drop them into the machine to be further transformed into a delicious drink or meal.

WASTE NOTHING!

The stems of all greens and herbs (except mint) can be juiced, so don't throw them out even if they're tough.

Whether you're using organic or conventional produce, be sure to wash everything very well in cool water before beginning. Even (and in some cases especially) organic produce can carry pathogens that should be rinsed off thoroughly. Put dark greens, lettuce leaves, and herbs in a deep bowl and cover them with cold water; swish them around to remove dirt and sand, then let them sit for a while so the residue sinks to the bottom of the bowl. Lift out the greens and drain well. Use a soft brush and running water to scrub whole fruits and vegetables that you don't intend to peel. Gently rinse whole berries in a colander under cool running water, letting them drain well.

If your greens are looking a little tired, mix them with filtered water or coconut water and blend. Then pour them into an ice cube tray and freeze. Add to your next smoothie for an extra dose of greens.

Prepping for the juicer: You'll need to do a bit of prep on some ingredients after you rinse or scrub them:

Ginger:	Some recipes specify peeled ginger. If so, peel it with a knife or vegetable peeler. In most cases, peeling is not necessary.
Citrus:	Peel or pare off the outer colored zest (save it for another use, if you'd like), but leave some of the white pith attached to the flesh: It contains nutrients that actually help your body absorb vitamin C. Citrus seeds also contain nutrients, so unless the bitterness they impart to the juice is too much for you, leave lemon seeds in. Larger grapefruit and orange seeds should be removed.
Mangos & stone fruits:	Remove the pits from tropical fruits, such as mangos, as well as apricots, peaches, and plums.
Watermelon:	Remove the outer green peel with a knife or vegetable peeler, but keep the white flesh near it. You can leave any seeds in, as they contain nutrients and don't change the flavor of the finished juice.
Cantaloupe & honeydew melon:	Remove the outer peel with a knife or vegetable peeler, and scrape out the inner seeds.

Most centrifugal juicers can handle fairly large pieces of fruits and vegetables—you can push a whole kale leaf, a whole stalk of celery, or a halved apple through with no problem. Mastication juicers require larger produce to be chopped into smaller pieces, about 2-inch chunks, so they can be dropped into the hopper. Check your juicer's manual for details about how to cut up produce for it.

Prepping for the blender: Obviously, you'll need to remove all but tender edible peels and seeds, and also roughly chop everything (and mince ingredients used in smaller quantities like ginger, fresh turmeric root, and garlic) before loading up your blender with produce. There's no need to peel or seed cucumbers, for example, but do remove the cores from apples. Pit and peel avocados. For a smoother smoothie, remove the tough stems and ribs from dark leafy greens like kale and collards—especially if you're not using a powerful high-end blender.

CHOOSING INGREDIENTS FOR FLAVOR AND HEALTH

There are many good reasons to buy organic produce whenever possible, but perhaps equally important is buying local. Every country has various rules governing the use of the term organic, some quite strict, some quite lax. Knowing the farms your produce comes from ensures an understanding of the processes and techniques they use. Organic produce is generally better for the environment, the farmer, the soil, the future, and, of course, you. From a health perspective, by choosing organic you should be limiting your intake of toxic pesticides and chemicals. Some research also shows that organically grown produce contains higher levels of nutrients.

It's true that organic produce can be difficult to find and more expensive than conventionally grown, so it's good to know that it doesn't have to be an all-or-nothing affair. You can prioritize your organic purchases based on current research: Whenever possible, buy organic apples, celery, cucumber, herbs, leafy greens, and berries. Many of these fruits and vegetables are known for having very high levels of pesticides when conventionally grown. Produce that you're going to peel, such as pineapple, melons, kiwi, avocado, and citrus, is less crucial. The website ewg.org contains an up-to-date list of the most and least contaminated produce in the United States and can be a helpful guide as you shop farmers' markets and grocery stores.

It probably goes without saying that in the fresh produce section you should look for fruits and vegetables with no signs of age or decay, no mold, and no wrinkles or soft spots where there shouldn't be. Use ripe specimens for the best flavor. Finally, don't neglect the frozen foods section of the grocery store, especially for smoothies; often frozen fruits and vegetables are of better quality than fresh produce because they're frozen just after harvesting, when they're at their peak.

VEGETABLES

Can you imagine eating a three-pound green salad? Didn't think so. But drinking it down in the form of a refreshing juice is no big deal. It's like a tasty multivitamin, full of enzymes, vitamins, and minerals, and because all the pulp and fiber is removed, the nutrients get absorbed quickly and you'll feel an instant boost of energy and vitality. The lack of fiber in juiced vegetables also gives your digestive system a break and is why a lot of people swear by juice cleanses: They can ingest a lot of nutrients while allowing the digestive system to rest. There's really no reason not to use just about any vegetable you like in a juice, and the recipes in this book make use of a mind-boggling variety, in all kinds of intriguing combinations. The following vegetables, however, are our standbys, the old favorites we turn to often to meet not only our energy and nutritional needs but also our desire for sustenance that's delicious and satisfying.

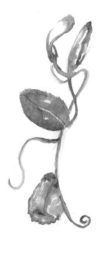

Leafy greens and herbs: Leafy greens—spinach, kale (Tuscan or curly), Swiss chard, collard greens, dandelion greens, and romaine lettuce, for example—are the foundation of green drinks, the ingredients that are nothing less than the reason green juices and smoothies exist. Greens and herbs are loaded with chlorophyll, which our body needs in order to support circulation and blood purification. All the dark, leafy greens are very high in calcium, magnesium, iron, potassium, phosphorous, zinc, and vitamins A, C, E, and K. These greens are also celebrated for their cancer-preventing benefits and ability to improve liver, gallbladder, and kidney functions. Leafy greens are great for people who experience a lot of congestion and mucus, and they provide a light, uplifting energy that also translates to how we might feel after ingesting them. Mix them with mild-tasting celery and cucumber, a little apple, lemon, and ginger and you've got yourself a nutritional powerhouse of a drink.

Tender herbs contribute distinctive flavors to your juices in addition to a nutrition boost. Cilantro (aka fresh coriander) is a great detoxifier, and parsley is high in vitamins A and C. Basil is an especially fragrant option and contains properties that relax the intestinal wall and relieve bloating and digestive discomfort.

Cucumber, celery, and fennel: Cucumber is a mainstay of fresh juice blends and smoothies because of its mild flavor and its high water content, which is cleansing and hydrating and helps bulk up the drink. It's cooling, too, of course, and is especially refreshing when paired with mint. Celery and faintly anise- or licorice-scented fennel bulbs are also cooling ingredients that are fabulous in juices.

Fennel has long been celebrated for its medicinal benefits— more specifically, its stomach-soothing abilities. It contains potent compounds that actually help relieve pain and spasms in the stomach. Celery is rich in minerals, especially calcium and potassium, so a juice loaded with celery works as a great electrolyte drink after a sweaty workout. It's also a great source of vitamin C, and has been shown to help relieve pain.

Carrots and beets: These naturally sweet root vegetables are ideal for adding a slightly sweet note to your juice blend. Carrots are high in beta-carotene, and beets are cell builders; together they support your liver and gallbladder. Beets are also celebrated for their blood-cleansing properties. They are high in folate, and their deep red color also indicates a good dose of antioxidants. Yams and sweet potatoes, other colorful, grounding root vegetables, make fun, unexpected additions to your juices, too.

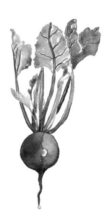

FRUITS

Sweet, juicy fruits are not only delicious but also an important part of a healthy diet. Just a little bit of fruit in the mix can take a bland juice or plain smoothie to another level. A word of caution is in order, however, especially if your body tends to react poorly to blood-sugar fluctuations or if you're trying to lose weight: Fruit sugar is still, well, sugar. If you consume too much fruit juice, which lacks the whole fruit's filling fiber, it can cause your blood-sugar to spike and then crash, resulting in a rollercoaster ride of sugar cravings, energy highs, and energy lows. Eating the whole fruit, as in a smoothie, is best, as the fiber will slow down the digestion and absorption of the sugar into your bloodstream and give you a steady stream of energy. Save most of your fruit intake for smoothies, and use it only in small amounts in juice.

Keeping a bag or two of sliced fruit or whole berries in the freezer makes it easy to throw just a few pieces at a time into a smoothie for a boost of antioxidants or sweetness and flavor.

Apples and pears: These are great fruits for juicing because they contain plenty of liquid without too much sugar. Apples are cleansing and can help stabilize blood sugar.

Berries: Raspberries, blueberries, blackberries, strawberries—all are great in both juices and smoothies. They're lower in sugar than most fruits, yet packed with antioxidants and anti-inflammatory benefits.

Tropical fruits and peaches: Used sparingly due to their high sugar content, fruits like pineapple, mangos, and peaches are a fun way to vary your juices and smoothies. Mangos are high in antioxidants that help protect the skin.

AROMATICS AND FLAVORINGS

Sure, you could just toss a combination of a few vegetables and maybe a fruit or two into the juicer, or blend up some frozen berries with a base of nut milk, a piece of avocado for body, and a spoonful of protein powder. You'd have a tasty, health-ful drink, no question. But the real fun of juicing and blend-ing drinks happens when you start adding small amounts of complementary—or contrasting—flavor elements. Many of these aromatics and enhancements, conveniently, have signifi-cant health benefits themselves. You'll find many ingredients in the recipes in this book that you might not have considered using in drinks before, from cacao nibs to orange blossom water, jalapeños to curry powder, fresh garlic to ground cayenne. Don't be shy with spice: Very often a sweet drink, for example, can benefit from a dose of heat or a savory coun-terpoint. A creamy, not-too-sweet smoothie can taste sweeter and more dessertlike with just a couple drops of pure vanilla extract or a dash of good cinnamon.

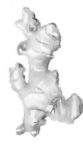

One of the most common aromatics used in these drinks is fresh ginger. It adds a little spice (or a lot, depending on how much you use), which helps to stimulate your taste buds.

Ginger increases circulation, it is anti-inflammatory, and it boosts your immune system. Fresh turmeric root, which is becoming more widely available in supermarket produce sections, is incredibly anti-inflammatory; it promotes healthy joints and adds a beautiful orange color to any juice, whether sweet or savory.

SMOOTHIE BASES

Nut and grain milks: Almond milk is deliciously creamy, thick, and still pretty low in calories. It contains a good amount of monounsaturated healthy fats and calcium. Try pistachio milk, hazelnut milk, rice milk, and coconut milk—all in unsweetened form, if possible. (See page 82 for how to make your own nut milks.)

Coconut water: Coconut water is often referred to as nature's sports drink. That's because it contains electrolytes, which are hydrating and prevent muscle cramping. You can easily use bottled juice, but if you can find fresh, young coconuts, snap them up, as fresh coconut water contains enzymes that help to detoxify and repair the body. (See page 122 for how to open one to harvest the water and coconut meat.) You can also sometimes find bottled coconut water that is raw and unpasteurized—in essence the same thing as fresh. Do check the label when buying bottled to make sure it is unsweetened; coconut water is naturally quite sweet and if it's good quality it shouldn't need any added sweeteners.

Avocado: Avocados are packed with healthy monounsaturated fats and oleic acid, and even some omega-3 fatty acids. These healthy fats help fight against heart disease and boost our good cholesterol. They also help fight inflammation and moisturize our skin from within. Smoothies with avocado have a creamy texture, similar to what you get from yogurt or banana, but without the sweetness.

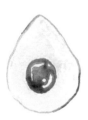

Dairy: Cow's milk lends a creamy texture to smoothies. It contains protein, fats, and vitamin D. However, it's best to use it with caution and know your body, as milk commonly causes digestive issues, skin breakouts, and mucus for those who cannot tolerate it well. Yogurt is a cultured dairy product that contains healthy bacteria, or probiotics. It contains a good amount of protein, and full-fat yogurt also contains some healthy vitamins and satisfying fats. Yogurt can be cooling for the body. No wonder lassis, yogurt-based smoothies, are so

If you're devising a "milk"-based smoothie, try adding some ground cinnamon, maca powder, and raw cacao powder. Cinnamon helps stabilize blood sugar, maca is a hormone balancer and good for the libido, and cacao is high in antioxidants and a powerful mood enhancer and energizer. If you want a sweeter-tasting smoothie, you can add a Medjool date or a little raw honey.

common in tropical and subtropical India, where cooling is especially welcome during or after a meal featuring spicy dishes.

SUPERFOODS

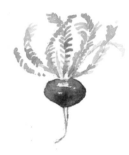

Maca: Maca is a South American root that is easily found in powder form. This adaptogenic superfood is known for its ability to increase energy, endurance, strength, and libido. No small promise! Maca also has hormone-balancing benefits, supporting the endocrine system, and can even offer some relief for perimenopause symptoms. By balancing hormones and boosting energy, maca can also have a positive effect on mood.

Acai: Acai is a berry from the Amazon packed with powerful antioxidants, helping fight free radicals and premature aging. This small dark purple berry also contains some fat, and when added to smoothies it adds a rich and creamy texture. These fats include the essentials—omega-3, -6, and -9—and so it has great heart-health and skin benefits, too. Acai can be found frozen, often in smoothie-ready packets, and as a powder. Both work great for boosting the nutritional value of your smoothies.

Goji berries: These little bright red berries from the Himalayas are packed with vitamin A as well as the two antioxidants lutein and zeaxanthin, which support good vision. Chinese medicine has utilized these potent berries for years to increase longevity and energy and boost memory. You can find goji berries in frozen, dried, juice, and powder forms. For smoothies, the powder is probably the most convenient way to go, especially if you don't have a powerful blender.

Cacao: Cacao has one of the highest antioxidant contents of any food. Look for it as whole beans, nibs, and unsweetened powder, ideally raw and not roasted. This superfood provides an energy boost, is a natural aphrodisiac, and helps elevate your mood due to its ability to increase serotonin levels. Cacao is also very high in magnesium, a mineral many of us are deficient in, as well as iron and calcium. The polyphenols found in cacao can even help lower bad cholesterol and benefit the heart. Both cacao nibs and unsweetened cacao powder work great in smoothies, especially creamy, milky ones.

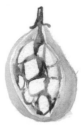

Baobab: Baobab is a fruit from an African tree with a delicious taste reminiscent of citrus sherbet. It's rich in antioxidants—more so than goji or acai—and does wonders for skin health. It's also fiber-rich, helping boost digestive health and keeping you feeling full for longer. Dried powdered baobab fruit is available in natural foods stores and online.

Bee pollen: These tiny golden balls of nutrient power are celebrated as the fountain of youth. Bee pollen contains both amino acids and vitamin B, making it a great supplement for vegans, who can have a harder time getting enough of these nutrients from other plant sources. It's also another great source of antioxidants and contains lecithin, which helps increase good cholesterol while lowering bad cholesterol.

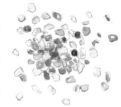

Probiotics: It turns out that the huge population of microbes and bacteria in our gut is responsible for many mechanisms in the body. These microbes and good bacteria are often referred to as probiotics, literally meaning "pro-life." Beyond boosting and regulating digestion, they also aid in nutrient absorption, and communicate with and regulate the immune system. Without healthy gut flora, our immune system and digestion suffer and we can end up feeling bloated and gassy and be more susceptible to infections and weight gain. These healthy microbes also help protect our gut lining, and in that way protect us from food allergies and sensitivities. Good bacteria in the gut can even influence behavior and affect mood—this is often referred to as the gut-brain connection. Probiotics can be found in fermented foods and beverages such as kimchi, sauerkraut, kefir, and kvass. Probiotics are also available as a supplement, either in powder form or as capsules (simply open a capsule and empty the contents into your juice or smoothie).

GREENS POWDERS

There's a broad range of greens powders available on the market today, and most of them contain a similar blend of dried or dehydrated green grasses often blended with a bit of stevia or dried fruits and berries. Some also contain algae, sprouts, and digestive enzymes. It's an easy and convenient way to add more greens to your diet, and perfect for adding to smoothies for an extra nutrient boost. Green grasses are energizing and invigorating for the body and contain a variety of vitamins and minerals, and they can help the body detoxify due to their high chlorophyll content. Concentrated greens are a great way to boost the protein content in smoothies and juices. These powders tend to be very concentrated; a little goes a long way.

Grasses: Barley grass and wheatgrass, often referred to as cereal grasses, are common ingredients in greens powders.

They contain 20 percent protein and are rich in chlorophyll. These grasses also contain unique digestive enzymes, which help aid digestion and dissolve toxins in food. They have anti-inflammatory properties and strengthen body tissue.

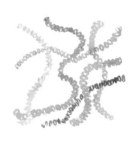

Blue-green micro-algae: Algae are aquatic plants and among the first primitive life forms on this planet; they contain large amounts of chlorophyll and are celebrated for their preventative, cleansing, and healing benefits. Both chlorella and spirulina are algae that contain a carotenoid called astaxanthin, which is one of the most powerful antioxidants that have been shown to protect the skin and eyes against UV radiation. Both spirulina and chlorella also contain a good amount of protein (spirulina contains more protein than chlorella), making them a useful supplement for vegans. Spirulina also contains GLA, a fatty acid that can boost weight loss.

E3 Live: E3 Live is made of wild freshwater blue-green algae that contains easily absorbed chlorophyll. Wild blue-green algae can be very beneficial during detox, as it helps cleanse your digestive tract. It is also believed to give a long-lasting energy boost and help with recovery from workouts.

CONCENTRATED PROTEIN SOURCES

Protein—found most abundantly in meat, eggs, and dairy but also in beans, lentils, nuts, seeds, whole grains, and leafy greens—is one of the body's most important building blocks, and what we need in order to restore and "build" muscles. There are eight amino acids that are essential to our body and that we need to get from our food. When a food contains all of these eight amino acids, we call it a complete protein. Our hormones are synthesized in our body from proteins, so it's important to get sufficient protein to keep a healthy hormone balance. Protein will also help you feel full longer and can therefore be helpful when trying to lose weight.

Adding a dose of protein to your smoothie or juice is a good way to make it into a drink that feels like a complete meal. Even if you're not using dairy in your drinks, it's easy to up the protein content with one or more of these additions.

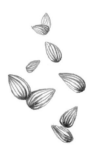

Almonds: Almonds, the most nutritious of all the nuts, in addition to being a good source of protein are high in healthy monounsaturated fats. They can stabilize blood sugar and lower the risk of diabetes, and lower cholesterol levels. Look for raw, unpasteurized almonds. Soaking them in cool water for a few hours or up to overnight before draining and blending them into a smoothie or other drink can make them more digestible. Use them in homemade almond nut milk (page 84).

Chia seeds: Tiny black chia seeds can absorb enormous quantities of water, and when soaked can swell to up to five times their size—their ability to hold on to water offers the body prolonged hydration and also helps you feel full longer, which aids weight loss. The seeds are high in fiber (which aids digestion and promotes regularity) and are the richest plant source of omega-3 fatty acids. They're essentially flavorless, so you can add them to anything.

Flaxseeds: Flaxseeds are another good source of protein, omega-3s, and fiber, and like chia seeds they have no discernible flavor of their own so they can be added to just about anything. It's best to buy fresh whole seeds and use a spice mill, mortar and pestle, or blender to grind them to a powder just before using them so the oils in the seeds stay fresh.

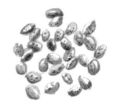

Protein powders: There is a mind-boggling array of protein powder supplements on the market, but most fall into a few broad categories (some commercial supplements may be composed of a combination of these). Check out the chart on page 22 to see which one is most appropriate for you.

Whey and pea protein powders are usually pure protein—that is, only the protein has been extracted from the dairy or the pea—so they contain minimal fat (usually around 2 grams per serving). Whey protein derived from grass-fed cows is always superior and will contain essential fatty acids and conjugated lineolic acid. Pea protein is completely plant based and vegan, it is free of any saturated or trans fats, and contains small amounts of unsaturated fat.

Hemp protein is usually just ground-up whole hemp seeds and therefore contains exactly the same nutrients, including omega-3 fatty acids, as hemp seeds.

Protein powders that contain soy are highly processed and not the health food some might believe them to be. Soy is one of the most genetically modified crops and a very common allergen, which a lot of people are sensitive to (even if they don't know it). The other issue with soy is that it contains antinutrients, including phytates, enzyme inhibitors, and goitrogens. It is also one of the foods that contains compounds that can mimic estrogen in the body. Instead of choosing protein

	Whey protein	Pea protein	Hemp protein
Description	derived from dairy	derived from peas	made from hemp seeds, often raw ground seeds, less processed than other protein powders
Ideal for	muscle builders; people recovering from injuries, adrenal fatigue, or auto-immune conditions; use following strenuous or heavy-lifting workouts	vegans and people with dairy allergies or sensitivities or digestive issues; pre- and post-workout	vegans and raw foodists
Protein	complete protein	complete protein	complete protein, but lower protein content
Fat	minimal	minimal	high fat content, ideal 3:1 omega-6 to -3 ratio
Other nutrients	provides amino acid glutamine, contains precursors of antioxi-dant glutathione	provides amino acid glutamine	high in zinc, iron, and magnesium
Possible benefits	helps regenerate intes-tinal flora for healthy gut and digestion; helps rebuild tissue; supports immune system; helps secretion and efficiency of insulin to regulate fat and carbohydrate metabolism	easily digested; assists with muscle recovery after workout	easily digested; good source of omega-3 and -6 in the right ratio; anti-inflammatory

powders containing soy, choose a pea-, rice-, or hemp- based protein, or a blend with a combination—all are vegan and generally very well tolerated. If you tolerate dairy, whey is another good protein source, especially for people recovering from illness or a tough workout.

No matter what protein source you choose, read the nutrition labels and the ingredients lists, as some protein powders may have added nutrients, flavors, sweeteners, and fats.

SWEETENERS

The best way to sweeten juices and smoothies is with real, whole foods. Fruits and vegetables are full of nutrients, are high in antioxidants, and contain fiber, which helps slow down the absorption of sugar into our bloodstream. Nature is pretty perfect and nutrients that are combined in one whole food also work together to optimize absorption and well-being for those who eat them. Fruits, and vegetables like beets and carrots, are often sweet enough to make a drink pleasant and enjoyable. Make sure to taste the drink before you add any other sweeteners, as it very likely won't need them at all! If you do choose to sweeten a drink, avoid highly refined sugars, highly refined agave nectar, and artificial sweeteners. The following are your best, most healthful options.

Raw honey: Raw honey has not been heated or processed in any way and therefore has all its beneficial nutrients intact, including antioxidants, minerals, vitamins, amino acids, and enzymes. Raw honey is also known for its antiviral and antibacterial properties, so it's no wonder it's such a good flu and cold fighter. Also, it's believed that eating raw honey that has been harvested in your local surroundings can significantly improve seasonal allergy symptoms.

Real maple syrup: Maple syrup is derived from the sap of the maple tree and is another great natural sweetener. It has a rich flavor and is packed with healthful minerals. One of those is manganese, which actually helps repair muscle and cell damage. Maple syrup also contains a good amount of antioxidants.

Coconut or palm sugar and syrup: Derived from the sweet juices of coconut palm sugar blossoms, coconut sugar and syrups contain twice the amount of iron, four times the magnesium, and more than ten times the amount of zinc than brown sugar, yet they have a relatively low glycemic index

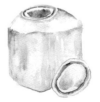

(35 compared to sugar's 68) so they don't cause such a high spike in blood-sugar levels. Coconut sugar is rich in enzymes, which help slow down its absorption into the bloodstream, another reason it's a great choice for anyone looking for a sweetener with low blood-sugar impact.

Yacon syrup: Yacon is a South American root, and the syrup made from it is rich in dietary fiber. Fiber acts as a prebiotic—that is, food for the good bacteria in our gut—and therefore supports healthy digestive function. Yacon syrup, like coconut sugar, is a low-glycemic sweetener. It's also rich in minerals and antioxidants. It's not the easiest sweetener to find and can be quite pricey, but if you can locate it (look for it online) and it fits in your budget, yacon syrup is an excellent sweetener.

Xylitol: Xylitol is a natural sugar alcohol found in the fibers of vegetables and fruits. It has very low impact on blood sugar and very few calories. Because it is a sugar alcohol, some people find that it irritates their gut and causes bloating or other discomforts. Others tolerate it well and love using it as a low-impact sweetener, so you might want to test it out for yourself and see how you like it. Xylitol has been found to inhibit oral bacteria, which is why you often find it in toothpaste, mints, and chewing gums.

Stevia: Stevia is a green plant with leaves that taste two to three hundred times sweeter than sugar, but with zero calories! No wonder this sweetener has taken off in the last few years, although it's been used for centuries in South America. Stevia does not feed yeast (or candida) or raise blood sugar. However, read the label before you buy: Many products that claim to be stevia in fact contain a lot of other additives and artificial sweeteners. Go for the purest kind you can find, or get a stevia plant for your garden!

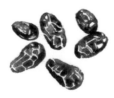

Medjool dates: Dates contain lots of fiber, which helps slow down sugar absorption. They are also high in antioxidants, vitamin B6, minerals, and tannins, so these sweet fruits are far from empty calories. Medjool dates are soft and chewy and have a rich caramel flavor that lends itself well to creamy smoothies and desserts.

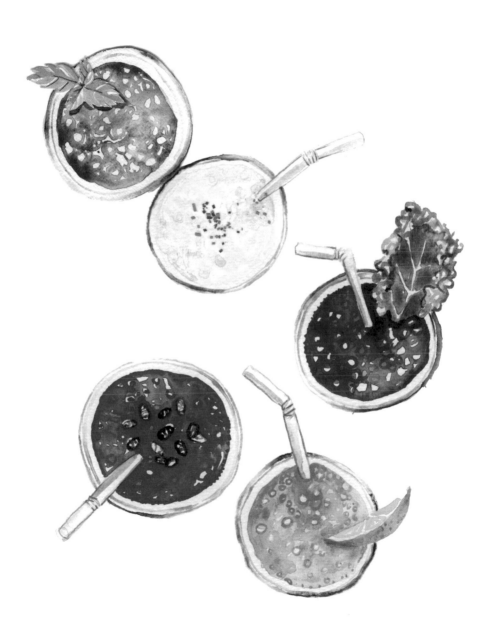

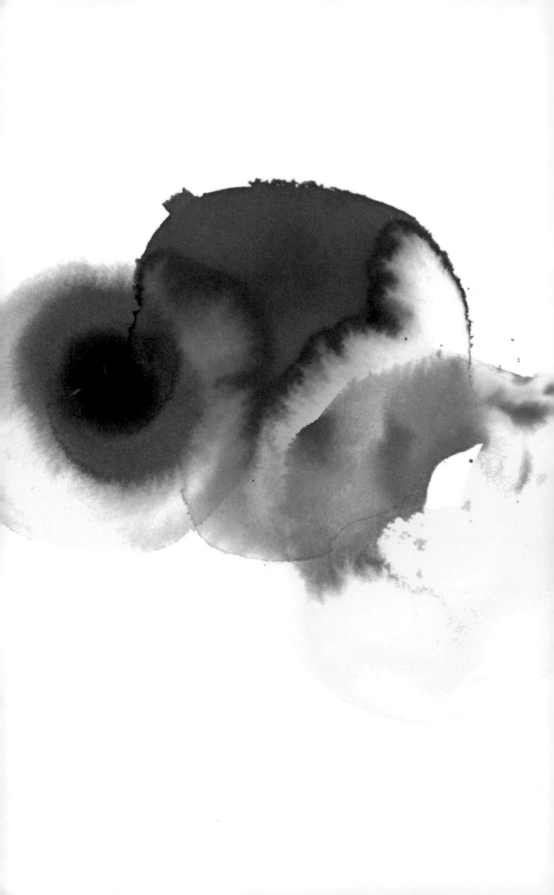

JUICES

Fresh-pressed juices are a fantastic way to add more nutritious fruit and vegetables to your diet—especially dark leafy greens, which work well in just about any blend of ingredients. If you've only ever had fresh orange juice, or a basic vegetable blend from the local juice stand, prepare to be wowed. From subtly sweet to bracing and savory, the following recipes will delight your senses, nourish your body, and stimulate your creative impulse: There's no doubt that these innovative combinations—most simple, some more elaborate and complex—will inspire you to come up with your own favorites based on your mood or specific nutritional needs. At the end of this chapter is a section of juice booster shots, which are intense, therapeutic, concentrated elixirs. It would probably be very difficult, even uncomfortable, to drink a tall glass of any one of these, but it's eminently doable in a small two-ounce portion. You get all the nutritional benefits concentrated in one quick throw-back shot. You've probably seen wheatgrass shots at your local health food store, but did you know that there are more nutrient-dense foods that lend themselves to being taken as shots? Try fresh ginger, berries, fresh turmeric root, and even garlic!

TIPS TO REMEMBER

- Always thoroughly wash fruits and vegetables prior to use.
- Core any apples or pears prior to use.
- Pit any stone fruits prior to use.
- Follow directions for your equipment. Centrifugal juicers can handle larger pieces of fruits and vegetables; masticating juicers require fruits and vegetables to be cut into smaller pieces.
- Volumes of final juices and smoothies can vary by more than 50 percent depending on size of fruits and vegetables used and type of juicer.
- Experiment! Once you've become familiar with the recipes, try swapping in different berries or greens or nut milks for different variations.

GREENE
The Juicery

Greens make your skin glow by nourishing your cells with minerals
and antioxidants. Aloe vera is healing to the skin and aids digestion,
and cucumber provides cooling hydration from the inside out.
The fennel in this mild, slightly tart juice adds a hint of licorice flavor.

. . . .

2 apples
2 inches (5 cm) cucumber
3 broccoli florets
1 bulb fennel
¾ lime, peeled
1 teaspoon aloe vera juice

Juice the apples, cucumber, broccoli, fennel, and lime,
then stir in the aloe vera juice. Serve immediately,
blended with ice, poured over ice cubes, or at room
temperature with no ice.

Makes one serving.

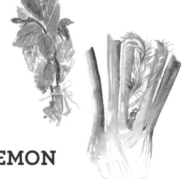

MINTY GREEN
FENNEL JUICE WITH LEMON
The Juicery

Fennel and mint are great for soothing an upset stomach. This cooling,
refreshing juice—with a shot of licorice flavor from the fennel—
is comforting, especially after a day of indulgence.

. . . .

1 green apple
1 bulb fennel, top cut off
½ lemon, peeled
2 kale leaves
5 mint leaves

Juice all the ingredients. Serve immediately, blended
with ice, poured over ice cubes, or at room temperature
with no ice.

Makes one serving.

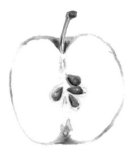

GUAVA APPLE CHILI JUICE
from Ananda in the Himalayas

Here's a metabolism-boosting juice with one unusual
fruity ingredient: guava. Guava contains more lycopene (an antioxidant)
than any other plant food and plenty of potassium.

2 guavas
½ small red apple
½ small green apple
About 1 teaspoon minced
   hot red chili, or to taste
½ lemon, peeled

Juice all the ingredients. Serve immediately, blended
with ice, poured over ice cubes, or at room temperature
with no ice.

Makes one serving.

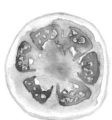

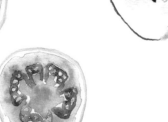

GREENWICH
The Juicery, The Marylebone Hotel

The Greenwich is a potent detox drink with a great antioxidant boost. Earthy beets are blood purifying and aid the liver and gallbladder in their detox work. This sweet, tangy juice should always be a part of any juice cleanse.

· ·

1½ apples
2 carrots
6 mint leaves
6 tablespoons (90 ml)
   beet juice (from ½ beet)
6 tablespoons (90 ml)
   pomegranate juice
   (from 1 cup/175 g
   pomegranate seeds)

Juice the apples, carrots, and mint, then stir in the beet and pomegranate juices. Serve immediately, blended with ice, poured over ice cubes, or at room temperature with no ice.

Makes one serving.

BEAUTY + THE BEET YEOTINI
from Michelle Ngoh, cofounder, Yeotown

A sweet and tart juice packed with beautifying and protective antioxidants. Beets and carrots used together like this can even help women with hormonal issues.

· ·

⅔ cup (100 g) blueberries
2 beets
2 carrots
1 apple
½ lemon, peeled
½ lime, peeled

Juice all the ingredients. Serve immediately, blended with ice, poured over ice cubes, or at room temperature with no ice.

Makes one serving.

BEET APPLE BLUSH

from Hala El-Shafie, founder, Nutrition Rocks

This beautiful and intensely colored juice has a multitude of health benefits, including nutrients that can help lower cholesterol, build blood, and boost athletic performance. And not only that, it tastes fabulous—sweet, with a bit of heat. If you can't find Pink Lady apples, which tend to arrive late in the season, try another super-sweet variety like Honeycrisp.

3 large beets
2 large Pink Lady apples
5 large carrots
1 inch (2.5 cm) fresh ginger

Juice all the ingredients. Serve immediately, blended with ice, poured over ice cubes, or at room temperature with no ice.

Makes one serving.

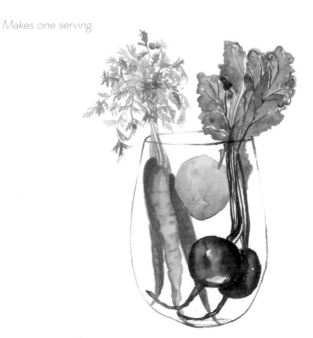

· ·

ULTIMATE ANTIOXIDANT JUICE
from Mathilde Thomas, founder, Caudalie

A beautiful red drink loaded with Caudalie's favorite antioxidant booster: grapes, which are rich in flavonoids and resveratrol. It turns out you don't have to drink red wine to reap the heart-healthy benefits of grapes! Any dark-colored variety of grape will work well here, including Concord.

· ·

1 beet
1 red or purple plum, pitted
¾ cup (115 g) red or purple grapes
¾ cup (115 g) mixed frozen berries

Juice the beet, plum, and grapes. Transfer to a blender, add the berries, and blend until smooth. Serve immediately, blended with ice, poured over ice cubes, or at room temperature with no ice.

Makes one serving.

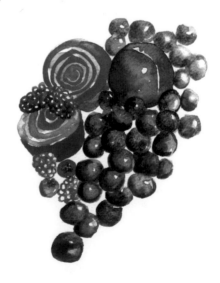

VIBRANT SKIN JUICE
The Juicery

Loaded with anti-inflammatory benefits and antioxidants to protect
the skin, this simple combination of sweet carrot and apple, spicy ginger,
tart lime, and juicy celery is delicious, too!

. . . .

2 carrots
4 stalks celery
2 (2-inch/5-cm) pieces
 fresh ginger
1 lime, peeled
1 apple

Juice all the ingredients. Serve immediately, blended
with ice, poured over ice cubes, or at room temperature
with no ice.

Makes one serving.

CARROT PEACH ORANGE
BASIL JUICE
The Juicery

This succulent, sweet juice is a real crowd-pleaser. Carrots are one of
the richest sources of the potent antioxidant beta-carotene, which also
gives them their signature bright orange color. Beta-carotene does
wonders for the skin and helps fight cancer.

. . . .

3 carrots
2 peaches, pitted
1 orange, peeled
5 basil leaves

Juice all the ingredients. Serve immediately, blended
with ice, poured over ice cubes, or at room temperature
with no ice.

Makes one serving.

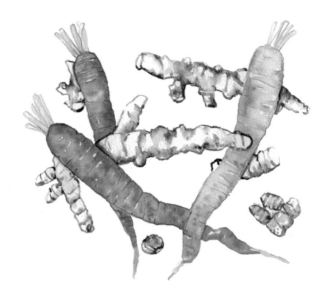

CARROT ORANGE TURMERIC JUICE
The Juicery

Turmeric is a potent inflammation fighter and helps regulate metabolism.
Beta-carotene from the carrots and vitamin C from the orange add
even more antioxidant power. You'll be fit for a fight and for healing after
a gulp of this earthy, sweet juice.

2 (2- to 3-inch/5- to
  7-cm) turmeric roots
3 carrots
2 oranges, peeled
5 mint leaves

Juice all the ingredients. Serve immediately, blended
with ice, poured over ice cubes, or at room temperature
with no ice.

Makes one serving.

BETA CLARITY JUICE
from Eve Persak, M.S., R.D., C.N.S.C.,
and Amanda Gale, COMO Shambhala

This beautifully creamy, sweet orange-colored juice can help soothe, soften, and clarify your skin. The carrots are known for their potential ability to improve vision, and papaya is rich in enzymes that can help repair damaged skin. The added coconut oil helps with nutrient absorption—especially of the fat-soluble vitamins.

10 carrots
½ red bell pepper
½ stalk celery
¼ bulb fennel
½ lemon, peeled
½ cup (70 g) papaya
  or mango
1 teaspoon coconut oil

Juice the carrots, bell pepper, celery, fennel, lemon, and papaya. Transfer to a blender and add the oil. Blend until creamy. Serve immediately, blended with ice, poured over ice cubes, or at room temperature with no ice.

Makes one serving.

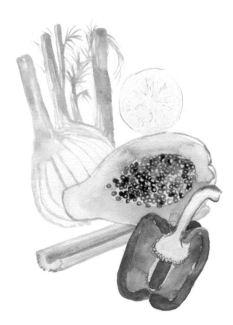

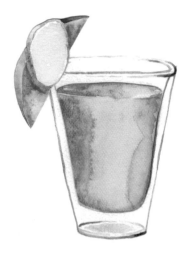

MERCER

The Juicery, The Kensington Hotel

This juice is packed with natural sweetness from fruits and vegetables, and will provide a nice boost of energy. The ginger is uplifting, a little spicy, and has anti-inflammatory benefits, while baobab is a potent antioxidant and multivitamin.

1 apple
4 carrots
5 long slices mango
1 inch (2.5 cm) fresh ginger

Recommended supplement:
1 teaspoon baobab

Juice the apple, carrots, mango, and ginger, then stir in the baobab. Serve immediately, blended with ice, poured over ice cubes, or at room temperature with no ice.

Makes one serving.

ANTIOXIDANT-RICH POMEGRANATE UPPER JUICE

from Shonali Sabherwal, macrobiotic nutritionist,
and chef, instructor, and founder, Soulfood India

Pomegranates have gotten a good rep lately—and with good reason!
The sweet-tart fruit is rich in vitamin B5 and antioxidants and is celebrated
for its positive impact on the skin. Chia seeds are considered a superfood,
packed with omega-3s, calcium, and fiber. Black salt—available at Indian
grocery stores—contains important trace minerals and its citrusy tang
will be especially welcome after a night of indulgence.

Seeds from 1 pomegranate
1 orange, peeled
1 teaspoon chia seeds
½ teaspoon black salt

Juice the pomegranate seeds and orange, then stir in the chia seeds and black salt. Serve blended with ice, poured over ice cubes, or at room temperature with no ice.

Makes one serving.

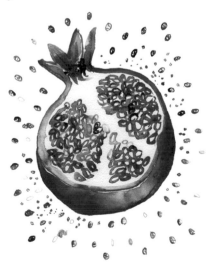

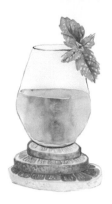

FIFTH AVENUE
The Juicery

This is the unofficial weight-loss booster in our lineup. Grapefruit (a well-known metabolism booster), apples (containing pectin, which works as a mild diuretic), and oranges (a great source of vitamin C) combine with mint for a refreshing citrusy tonic that's just slightly bitter from the grapefruit.

. . . .

1 apple
½ grapefruit, peeled
2 oranges, peeled
1 lime, peeled
5 mint leaves

Juice all the ingredients. Serve immediately, blended with ice, poured over ice cubes, or at room temperature with no ice.

Makes one serving.

HANGOVER HELPER
The Juicery

Some mornings are just a little tougher than others. Start them off right with a hydrating juice packed with anti-inflammatory ginger and liver-boosting lemon and beets. The comforting sweetness and citrusy tang, plus the bite of fresh ginger, will be especially welcome after a night of indulgence.

. . . .

2 oranges, peeled
1 beet
2 stalks celery
2 inches (5 cm) fresh ginger
½ lemon, peeled
1 teaspoon aloe vera juice

Juice the oranges, beet, celery, ginger, and lemon, then stir in the aloe vera juice. Serve immediately, blended with ice, poured over ice cubes, or at room temperature with no ice.

Makes one serving.

MORNING FLUSH DRINK
from Kay Kay Clivio, lead trainer, Pure Yoga, New York

This is a potent morning drink intended to help flush out toxins.
With both ginger and garlic, this spicy drink is intended for the more
experienced and adventurous juicers out there. You know who you are.

2 oranges, peeled
3 cloves garlic
1 inch (2.5 cm) fresh ginger
1 to 2 tablespoons cold-
  pressed extra-virgin
  olive oil
1⅓ cups (320 ml) filtered
  water

Juice the oranges, garlic, and ginger, then stir in the
oil and water. Serve blended with ice, poured over ice
cubes, or at room temperature with no ice.

Makes one serving.

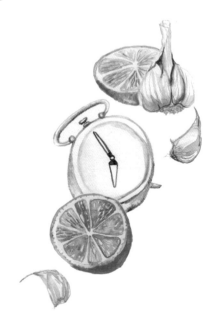

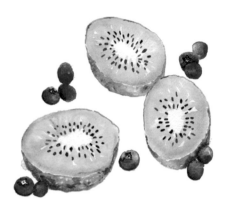

KIWI BLUEBERRY COOLER
The Juicery

Blueberries are high in antioxidants and low in sugar, kiwi adds
a boost of immune-system-supporting vitamin C, and cucumber
provides plenty of hydration. Barely sweet, a little tart, and fragrant
with fresh basil, this cooler won't weigh you down.

2 kiwi fruit, peeled
1⅔ cups (245 g) blueberries
2 stalks celery
12 inches (30 cm) cucumber
5 basil leaves

Juice all the ingredients. Serve immediately, blended
with ice, poured over ice cubes, or at room temperature
with no ice.

Makes one serving.

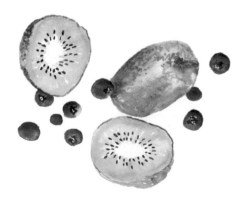

TATA'S HYDRATING JUICE

from Tata Harper, founder, Tata Harper Skincare

Sweet and citrusy, with a subtle floral fragrance, this juice is best when made with summer-ripe strawberries, melon (any variety will do), and apricots.

. . . .

12 inches (30 cm) cucumber
4 strawberries
1 carrot
½ cup (80 g) melon
3 to 4 apricots, pitted
½ orange, peeled
¼ cup (60 ml) unsweetened
   coconut water
1 tablespoon rosewater

Juice the cucumber, strawberries, carrot, melon, apricots, and orange, then stir in the coconut water and rosewater. Serve immediately, blended with ice, poured over ice cubes, or at room temperature with no ice.

Makes one serving.

TATA'S SKIN-CLEANSING JUICE

from Tata Harper, founder, Tata Harper Skincare

Here you get the best of both worlds with a cleansing juice that helps clear up the skin and boost it with hydration from within. Cucumber contains silica, which is important for collagen formation, and orange is rich in vitamin C, which helps counteract the wrinkle formation in the skin. Aloe vera is calming and cleansing, and raw honey is antibacterial. Who doesn't want well-hydrated, plump, dewy, and younger-looking skin?

. . . .

½ stalk celery
2 inches (5 cm) cucumber
2 apples
2 oranges, peeled
2 tablespoons raw honey
1 tablespoon aloe vera juice
1 tablespoon orange
   blossom water
⅓ cup (80 ml) unsweetened
   coconut water

Juice the celery, cucumber, apples, and oranges, then stir in the honey, aloe vera juice, and orange blossom and coconut waters. Serve immediately, blended with ice, poured over ice cubes, or at room temperature with no ice.

Makes one serving.

WHOLE FOOD JUICE

from Moises Mehl, raw food chef, nood food

The silica and sulfur in cucumbers supports healthy hair growth,
while kale's high antioxidant content can boost immunity.
Spirulina, a complete protein, has been shown to aid the production
of serotonin (aka "happy juice") while also promoting detoxification.
This is a mild, somewhat grassy juice; it makes an excellent
after-yoga replenisher.

. . . .

4 inches (10 cm) cucumber
2 stalks celery
2 cups (80 g) kale
½ apple

Recommended supplement:
½ teaspoon spirulina powder

Juice the cucumber, celery, kale, and apple, then stir
in the spirulina. Serve immediately, blended with ice,
poured over ice cubes, or at room temperature with
no ice.

Makes one serving.

FENNEL CUCUMBER JUICE

from Abigail James, international facialist
and well-being expert

This juice makes a refreshingly green and clean morning cocktail.
Fennel adds a delicious licorice flavor.

. . . .

9 inches (23 cm) cucumber
1 lemon, peeled
½ bulb fennel
2 inches (5 cm) fresh ginger
½ cup (20 g) spinach
4 to 6 mint leaves

Juice all the ingredients. Serve immediately, blended
with ice, poured over ice cubes, or at room temperature
with no ice.

Makes one serving.

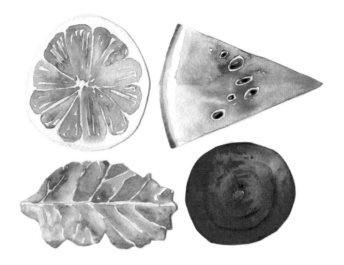

JUICAGRA

from Dr. Naveen Kella, director and cofounder of
Urology & Prostate Institute, Division of Oncology San Antonio

This drink was created by Dr. Kella, a urologist, to help maximize
not only your overall health but specifically your sexual health.
Kale provides an energy boost, watermelon can help improve blood flow,
and beets help boost your stamina. Okay, then!

1 cup (150 g) watermelon
3 cups (120 g) kale
1 small beet
½ ruby red grapefruit, peeled

Juice all the ingredients. Serve immediately, blended
with ice, poured over ice cubes, or at room temperature
with no ice.

Makes one serving.

SUMMER COOLER
The Juicery

Watermelon is the ultimate summer food: hydrating and cooling,
and a mild diuretic. A little dose of fresh mint adds some additional
chill to this refreshing treat.

· ·

2½ cups (380 g) watermelon
1⅓ cups (210 g) cantaloupe
1 cup (20 g) parsley
5 mint leaves

Juice all the ingredients. Serve immediately, blended
with ice, poured over ice cubes, or at room temperature
with no ice.

Makes one serving.

HONEY HYDRATOR
The Juicery

Honeydew and aloe vera are fantastic for the skin. Parsley is
extremely nutritious, with more vitamin C, gram for gram, than any citrus,
and is strengthening for our overworked adrenal glands. The grassy flavor
of parsley is nicely complemented here by sweet melon and tangy lime.

· ·

3 stalks celery
1¾ cups (300 g) honeydew
   melon
½ cup (20 g) parsley
½ lime, peeled
1 teaspoon aloe vera juice

Juice the celery, melon, parsley, and lime, then stir in
the aloe vera juice. Serve immediately, blended with
ice, poured over ice cubes, or at room temperature with
no ice.

Makes one serving.

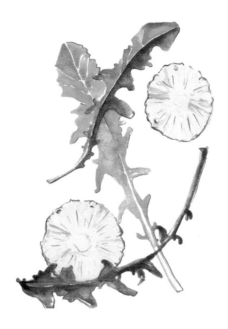

SPICY DANDELION PINEAPPLE JUICE
from Christina Agnew and Clare Neill,
cofounders, Radiance

Dandelion (yes, it's a weed, but so much more) supports healthy liver function and is packed with minerals and vitamins. Combined with the sweetness of pineapple and the heat of jalapeño, this astringent green might just become your newest obsession.

1 cup (40 g) dandelion greens
1½ cups (145 g) pineapple
1 jalapeño, seeded
Strips of lime zest

Juice the dandelion greens, pineapple, and jalapeño. Serve immediately, blended with ice, poured over ice cubes, or at room temperature with no ice, garnished with lime zest.

Makes one serving.

GLOW AND TELL

from Christina Agnew and Clare Neill,
cofounders, Radiance

In-season watermelon contains the antioxidant lycopene, which is
great for your skin. Along with a few sprigs of mint, it's also cooling
and refreshing—just what you need in the hot summer months.
Ginger is good for digestion, which is important even when drinking juice.
A small piece of beet adds a beautiful color.

6 inches (15 cm) cucumber
2½ cups (380 g) watermelon
Small handful mint leaves
3 teaspoons minced fresh
　ginger
1 lime, peeled
2 apples
¼ beet

Juice all the ingredients. Serve immediately, blended
with ice, poured over ice cubes, or at room temperature
with no ice.

Makes one serving.

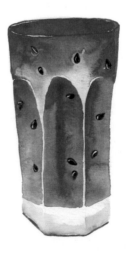

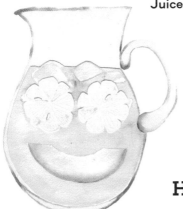

HAPPY JUICE
The Juicery

St. John's wort is used to treat depression and can help elevate your mood. Added to this sweet and sour, slightly peppery juice, it should be enough to at least bring a smile to your face.

½ honeydew melon
1 Bosc pear
1 green apple
½ lemon, peeled
1 (2- to 3-inch/5- to 7-cm) turmeric root
¼ teaspoon St. John's wort extract

Juice all the ingredients, then stir in the St. John's wort extract. Serve immediately, blended with ice, poured over ice cubes, or at room temperature with no ice.

Makes one serving.

PINEAPPLE AND GINGER LIFTER
from Ananda in the Himalayas

Feel uplifted with a boost of fiery ginger, cooling mint, and sweetly delicious pineapple loaded with enzymes to aid digestion and detoxification.

1½ cups (250 g) pineapple
1 inch (2.5 cm) fresh ginger
5 mint leaves

Juice all the ingredients. Serve immediately, blended with ice, poured over ice cubes, or at room temperature with no ice.

Makes one serving.

RASPBERRY GREEN FLAX JUICE
The Juicery

Raspberries, those sweet-and-sour stars of summer, are not only delicious but also have blood purifying benefits as well. And flaxseeds are high in omega-3 fatty acids and celebrated for their anti-inflammatory benefits. Fresh turmeric root and collard greens add a pungent note that highlights but doesn't overwhelm the delicate flavor of the berries.

3 cups (370 g) raspberries
1½ cups (60 g) collard
  greens
1 (2- to 3-inch/5- to 7-cm)
  turmeric root
2 tablespoons flaxseeds
½ teaspoon ground
  cinnamon

Juice the raspberries, collard greens, and turmeric. Strain through a sieve. Transfer to a blender, add the flaxseeds and blend, then stir in the cinnamon. Serve immediately, blended with ice, poured over ice cubes, or at room temperature with no ice.

Makes one serving.

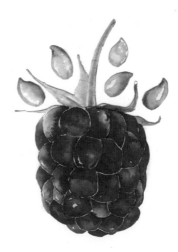

SPICY SPINACH
CUCUMBER LIME JUICE
The Juicery

A great detox juice, this one features cilantro, a potent chelator
of heavy metals. Cucumber is nice and cooling for the body, and lime
benefits the liver—our main detoxing organ.

· ·

½ cup (8 g) cilantro
1 cup (40 g) spinach
12 inches (30 cm) cucumber
1 lime, peeled

Juice all the ingredients. Serve immediately, blended
with ice, poured over ice cubes, or at room temperature
with no ice.

Makes one serving.

TANGY GREENS
The Juicery

A nicely tart and refreshing juice that will perk you up and help
your body detox with apples, greens, and herbs.

· ·

2 apples
3 limes, peeled, or more
   to taste
¼ cup (10 g) kale
¼ cup (10 g) spinach
2 tablespoons parsley
1 stalk celery

Juice all the ingredients. Serve immediately, blended
with ice, poured over ice cubes, or at room temperature
with no ice.

Makes one serving.

SWEET AND SPICY JUICE
The Juicery

Lots of chlorophyll-boosting greens and refreshing citrus make this
a delicious and nutritious juice any time of day. It's great for the skin
and helps boost immunity, too. Spicy with ginger, it would be
especially warming in wintertime.

. . . .

2¾ cups (100 g) green
   Swiss chard
½ cup (40 g) arugula
1 Bosc pear
1 orange, peeled
1 lime, peeled
1 inch (2.5 cm) fresh ginger

Juice all the ingredients. Serve immediately, blended
with ice, poured over ice cubes, or at room temperature
with no ice.

Makes one serving.

CLEAN GREEN SPINACH
from Dr. Alejandro Junger, medical director and creator,
the Clean Program

Every ingredient in this juice is hydrating, cleansing, and nourishing.
It's great to incorporate slightly bitter foods like kale into your diet to aid in
overall digestion, help keep blood sugar stable, and curb sugar cravings.

. . . .

1 cup (40 g) kale
2 cups (80 g) spinach
4 stalks celery
1 small carrot
1 inch (2.5 cm) fresh ginger
½ lemon, peeled

Juice all the ingredients. Serve immediately, blended
with ice, poured over ice cubes, or at room temperature
with no ice.

Makes one serving.

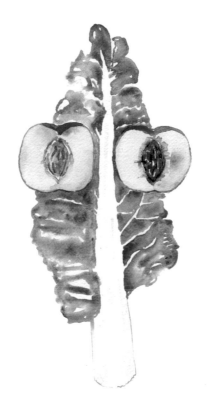

PEACHES 'N' GREEN
The Juicery

Peaches are a summery treat and are said to even help limit perspiration on hot summer days. Combined with greens and refreshing basil, sweet ripe peaches make a not-too-sweet green juice.

1¾ cups (70 g) spinach
1¾ cups (70 g) Swiss chard
2 peaches, pitted
5 basil leaves

Juice all the ingredients. Serve immediately, blended with ice, poured over ice cubes, or at room temperature with no ice.

Makes one serving.

GREEN GETS GORGEOUS YEOTINI

from Michelle Ngoh, cofounder, Yeotown

Greens are great for promoting healthy, glowing skin. This juice
is loaded with mineral-rich kale and spinach as well as vitamin C from
lemon and lime. Gently cleansing and delicious, this drink, well,
makes you gorgeous—inside and out!

Handful spinach
Handful kale
1 small bunch parsley
6 inches (15 cm) cucumber
4 stalks celery
1 apple
½ lemon, peeled
½ lime, peeled

Juice all the ingredients. Serve immediately, blended
with ice, poured over ice cubes, or at room temperature
with no ice.

Makes one serving.

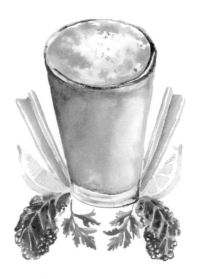

VERY GREEN JUICE

from Mark Zeitouni, executive chef,
Standard Hotel, Miami

Romaine lettuce is often overlooked as a nutritious leafy green,
but did you know this mild lettuce is 17 percent protein and contains more
vitamin C, gram for gram, than an orange? This juice is completely free
of fruit—no sugar here, just all good greens!

. . . .

1 head romaine lettuce
1 cucumber
2 stalks celery
1½ kale leaves
½ cup (15 g) tightly packed
   parsley
1 cup (40 g) spinach

Juice all the ingredients. Serve immediately,
blended with ice, poured over ice cubes, or at
room temperature with no ice, or store in a covered
container in the refrigerator for up to 27 hours.

Makes one serving.

GRACEFUL GREENS

from Amelia Freer, nutritional therapist and founder,
Freer Nutrition

This juice is not only refreshingly cooling, but it also helps hydrate
you and replenish your body after a sweaty day at the beach or in the gym.

. . . .

1 cup (40 g) spinach or kale
1 pear
6 inches (15 cm) cucumber
1 lime, peeled
2 sprigs parsley
2 sprigs mint, stemmed
Unsweetened coconut water

Juice the spinach, pear, cucumber, lime, parsley,
and mint, then stir in coconut water to taste. Serve
immediately, blended with ice, poured over ice cubes,
or at room temperature with no ice.

Makes one serving.

CLEAN GREEN CILANTRO

from Dr. Alejandro Junger, medical director and creator,
the Clean Program

Did you know that cilantro can actually help chelate out
heavy metals from your body? Now that is one potent herb!
This juice will help your body do its detoxing thing while also
boosting you up with lots of energizing nutrients.

· ·

1 cup (40 g) spinach
Handful fresh cilantro
12 inches (30 cm) cucumber
1 lemon, peeled
Filtered water

Juice the spinach, cilantro, cucumber, and lemon, then
stir in water to taste. Serve immediately, blended with
ice, poured over ice cubes, or at room temperature with
no ice.

Makes one serving.

GO GREEN JUICE

from Saimaa Miller, naturopath and author,
Aussie Body Diet and Detox Plan, Aussie Body Diet Pty. Ltd.

Kiwi is a vitamin C powerhouse with an unexpected and delicious
taste. This juice is loaded with minerals, antioxidants, and flavor.

· ·

1 kiwi
½ cup (20 g) spinach
3 large kale leaves
1 carrot
1 lime, peeled
A few sprigs cilantro
1 green apple

Juice all the ingredients. Serve immediately, blended
with ice, poured over ice cubes, or at room temperature
with no ice.

Makes one serving.

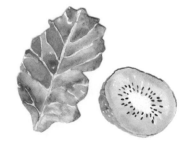

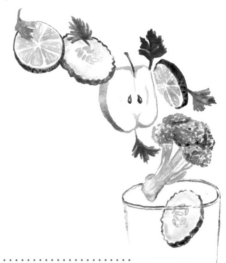

CLEAN GREEN JUICE

from Christina Agnew and Clare Neill,
cofounders, Radiance

With its slightly sweet-tart flavor profile, you'd be surprised
how low in fruit this juice is—a great option if you want to avoid spiking
your blood sugar. Cucumber is high in silica and helps build healthy
connective tissue. Parsley, broccoli, and kale are rich in the antioxidants
vitamins C and A, which help protect our skin cells.

12 inches (30 cm) cucumber
2 apples
½ small head broccoli,
 including the stalk
1 cup (50 g) tightly packed
 kale
½ cup (15 g) loosely packed
 parsley
1 lime, peeled

Juice all the ingredients. Serve immediately, blended
with ice, poured over ice cubes, or at room temperature
with no ice.

Makes one serving.

· ·

THE HANGOVER HELPER: SUPER GREEN JUICE

from Susan Blum, M.D., director, Blum Center for Health
in Rye Brook, NY; author, *The Immune System Recovery Plan*

This tart green juice is a great way to support liver detoxification
after a night out on the town, while also soothing your stomach.
The ginger aids in digestion and helps treat nausea, while cucumbers
and kale are a rich source of antioxidants, which help perk up
all the cells in your body.

· ·

5 kale leaves
1 stalk celery
1 green apple
6 inches (15 cm) cucumber
½ lemon, peeled
1 tablespoon chopped
 fresh ginger
2 tablespoons parsley

Juice all the ingredients. Serve immediately, blended
with ice, poured over ice cubes, or at room temperature
with no ice.

Makes one serving.

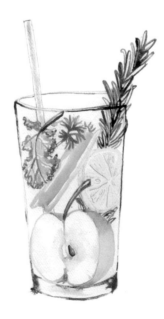

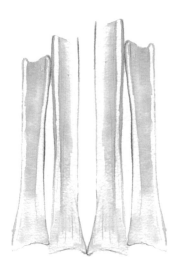

KALE-ADE

from Dr. Andrew Weil, True Kitchen

A fantastic green juice that is sure to become an everyday favorite—
hydrating, alkalizing, and refreshing, with a hint of spice.

4 stalks celery
12 inches (30 cm) cucumber, peeled
1 Gala or Fuji apple
10 kale leaves
4 inches (10 cm) fresh ginger, peeled
1 lemon, peeled and seeded

Juice all the ingredients. Serve immediately, blended with ice, poured over ice cubes, or at room temperature with no ice.

Makes one serving.

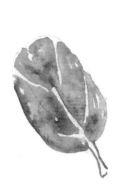

. . . .

BACKSTAGE
The Juicery

This juice is the backstage secret! Loaded with hydrating, replenishing, and energizing ingredients, it's a juice that makes you fit for fight. Spinach is loaded with iron and calcium, and the cucumber is cooling and hydrating to help you keep calm and carry on.

. . . .

2 cups (80 g) spinach
1 pear
5 basil leaves
12 inches (30 cm) cucumber
½ cup (120 ml) unsweetened
   coconut water
2 tablespoons yuzu juice

Juice the spinach, pear, basil, and cucumber, then stir in the coconut water and yuzu juice. Serve immediately, blended with ice, poured over ice cubes, or at room temperature with no ice.

Makes one serving.

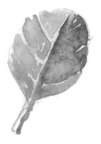

CLEAN AND LEAN GREENS
from Eve Persak, M.S., R.D., C.N.S.C.,
and Amanda Gale, COMO Shambhala

A delicious juice that helps build lean muscle, boosts energy and immunity, and bolsters the detoxification systems. This is one of the primary juices used in COMO Shambhala's cleanse program. Fresh juices are blended with sunflower seeds and nuts for a creamy mouthfeel, and spirulina gives the drink a vaguely saline quality.

2 apples
1 stalk celery
½ bulb fennel
6 inches (15 cm) cucumber
½ cup (20 g) spinach
½ green bell pepper
1 tablespoon raw, shelled
  sunflower seeds
1 tablespoon macadamia nuts

Recommended supplement:
1 teaspoon spirulina powder

Juice the apples, celery, fennel, cucumber, spinach, and bell pepper. Transfer to a blender and add the sunflower seeds, macadamia nuts, and spirulina, if using; blend until smooth. Serve immediately, blended with ice, poured over ice cubes, or at room temperature with no ice.

Makes one serving.

CLEANSING COCKTAIL
from Chiva-Som International Health Resort

Earthy, sweet beets are blood-purifying, and ginger adds
a nice kick with anti-inflammatory benefits.

. . . .

1½ cups (12 inches / 30 cm)
    cucumber
1½ cups (190 g) red apple
1½ cups (190 g) carrots
1½ cups (180 g) beets
1 teaspoon chopped fresh
    ginger

Juice all the ingredients. Serve immediately, blended
with ice, poured over ice cubes, or at room temperature
with no ice.

Makes one serving.

GET GROUNDED JUICE
The Juicery

Roots bring us closer to the earth and have what we call "grounding"
abilities. If you're feeling stressed or a bit scattered, this is the juice for you.
Dandelion greens are available in most good markets, but if your
lawn is all-natural you could also forage them straight from the yard—
pick smaller leaves, just before the yellow blossoms appear.

. . . .

1⅓ cups (60 g) dandelion
    greens
1 beet
5 to 6 red radishes (no tops)
2 carrots
2 inches (5 cm) fresh ginger

Juice all the ingredients. Serve immediately, blended
with ice, poured over ice cubes, or at room temperature
with no ice.

Makes one serving.

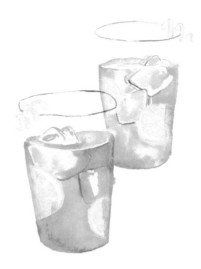

GINGER LEMON LOTUS JUICE

The Juicery

Savory lemonades are fairly common in Southeast Asia,
and this spicy green one is sure to perk you up on a sluggish day.

3 stalks celery
1 cup (40 g) spinach
2 lemons, zest peeled
  (for garnish)
2 inches (5 cm) fresh ginger
Pinch sea salt

Juice the celery, spinach, lemons, and ginger, then stir in the salt. Serve immediately, blended with ice, poured over ice cubes, or at room temperature with no ice, and with shaved lemon peels for garnish.

Makes one serving.

BRAIN FOOD SMOOTHIE
The Juicery

This is a real superfood blend, with maca for its memory-boosting benefits, avocado for its healthy fats, and bee pollen and E3 Live, an edible form of blue-green algae, for a real energy boost. The sweet grapes and banana make this subtly green smoothie go down easy.

2 cups (80 g) kale
1⅔ cups (250 g) stemmed
  grapes
12 inches (30 cm) cucumber
½ avocado
1 banana

Recommended supplements:
1 teaspoon bee pollen
1 teaspoon maca
1 tablespoon E3 Live

Juice the kale, grapes, cucumber, avocado, and banana, then stir in the supplements. Serve immediately, blended with ice, poured over ice cubes, or at room temperature with no ice.

Makes one serving.

LIVER-CLEANSING JUICE

from Michelle Roques-O'Neil, aromatherapist, healer,
spiritual life coach, and natural perfumer

This mildly sweet juice is packed full of vegetables and fruits
to boost your liver function and help your body detoxify. It's rich
in protein, calcium, omega-3s, iron, and vitamin C.

6 inches (15 cm) cucumber
½ beet
2 carrots
1 head romaine lettuce
2 stalks celery
1 inch (2.5 cm) fresh ginger
½ green apple
½ pink grapefruit, peeled
10 mint leaves

Recommended supplement:
1 teaspoon wheatgrass
    powder

Juice all the ingredients, then stir in the wheatgrass
powder. Serve immediately, blended with ice, poured
over ice cubes, or at room temperature with no ice.

Makes one serving.

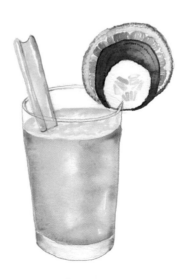

JOE'S MEAN GREEN JUICE
from Joe Cross, author, *Reboot with Joe Juice Diet;*
founder, Reboot with Joe

This might just become a trusted staple in your new juicy lifestyle.
With a little sweetness and a touch of spice, plus tons of green
power from kale, it's delicious as well as nutritious.

· ·

12 inches (30 cm) cucumber
4 stalks celery
2 apples
6 to 8 kale leaves
½ lemon, peeled
1 tablespoon chopped fresh
   ginger

Juice all the ingredients. Serve immediately, blended with ice, poured over ice cubes, or at room temperature with no ice.

Makes one serving.

DALTON'S RED JUICE
from Dalton Wong, Twenty Two Training

Sweet beet juice is not only good for detoxification and your liver—
it also helps increase your stamina and helps the body respond better
to exercise. The coconut water adds potassium and electrolytes.

· ·

1 cup (40 g) spinach
3 small beets
½ red bell pepper
1 cup (240 ml) unsweetened
   coconut water

Juice the spinach, beets, and bell pepper, then stir in the coconut water. Serve immediately, blended with ice, poured over ice cubes, or at room temperature with no ice.

Makes one serving.

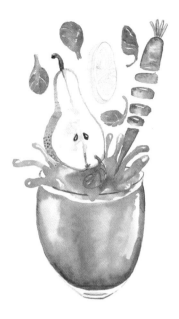

HYDRATOR JUICE
from Dalton Wong, Twenty Two Training

A hydrating and antioxidant-packed juice for every day.
Coconut water adds a fun and refreshing twist to this juice and
provides you with plenty of replenishing electrolytes.

½ pear
1 cup (40 g) spinach
½ red bell pepper
1 carrot
½ lemon, peeled
½ cup (120 ml) unsweetened
   coconut water

Juice the pear, spinach, bell pepper, carrot, and lemon,
then stir in the coconut water. Serve immediately,
blended with ice, poured over ice cubes, or at room
temperature with no ice.

Makes one serving.

VIBRANT

The Juicery, The Marylebone Hotel

Inspired by famed London florist Nikki Tibbles, from Wild at Heart, this juice is loaded with colorful, beauty-fortifying foods. The citrus offers vitamin C, an antioxidant that helps boost the immune system and has antiaging benefits for the skin. Berries are also full of antioxidants and help protect against damage to our cells. The beta-carotene in mango is also a great antioxidant that helps boost collagen production in the skin. Rosewater and orange blossom water add a delicious taste, and their aromas are nice and calming.

½ cup (60 g) raspberries
½ cup (60 g) strawberries, plus 1 for garnish
⅔ cup (100 g) mango
¼ lemon, peeled
¼ lime, peeled
¾ cup (180 ml) unsweetened coconut water
1 teaspoon rosewater
½ teaspoon orange blossom water

Juice the raspberries and strawberries and strain through a fine-mesh sieve. Juice the mango, lemon, and lime and stir into the berry juices. Stir in the coconut water, rosewater, and orange blossom water. Serve over ice and garnish with a fresh strawberry.

Makes one serving.

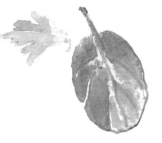

SPICY GREENS SHOT
The Juicery

This bright green shot is rich in chlorophyll, which is energizing and cleansing. Spinach and kale, the two main ingredients, also contain iron and calcium! The lemon and ginger aid with digestion and detoxification, and provide a tart, spicy counterpoint to the slightly bitter greens.

· ·

1 kale leaf
5 spinach leaves
1 sprig cilantro
1 inch (2.5 cm) fresh ginger
¼ lemon, peeled

Juice all the ingredients. Serve immediately.

Makes one serving.

SEA BUCKTHORN SHOT
The Juicery

Sea buckthorn berries are loaded with nutrients for the skin and are one of the most concentrated sources of vitamin C. Bottoms up!

· ·

6 tablespoons (60 g)
  sea buckthorn berries,
  fresh or frozen
4 teaspoons almond milk,
  or to taste
Raw honey to taste

Juice the berries. Stir in almond milk and honey to taste. Serve immediately.

Makes one serving.

LEMON GINGER CAYENNE SHOT
The Juicery

Feel a cold coming on? This spicy shot provides a boost
of vitamin C for your immune system. Ginger helps fight
inflammation, and cayenne helps loosen mucus.

. . . .

½ lemon, peeled
1 inch (2.5 cm) fresh ginger
Pinch ground cayenne

Juice the lemon and ginger and stir in the cayenne.
Serve immediately.

Makes one serving.

ELIXIR GREENWICH GINSENG
from Santosh Jori, executive chef, Westin Hotels & Resorts,
The Westin Beijing Financial Street

Packed with antioxidants, vitamin C for immune support, and beta-carotene
for the skin, this revitalizing juice is great for road warriors in need
of a boost. Ginseng is traditionally known for increasing energy and
supporting overall well-being. Yes, please!

. . . .

1½ oranges, peeled
1 green apple
1 carrot
¼ teaspoon ginseng
   powder
Mixed berries and lemon
   slice for garnish

Juice the oranges, apple, and carrot, then stir in the
ginseng. Serve immediately, blended with ice, poured
over ice cubes, or at room temperature with no ice,
garnished with berries and a lemon slice.

Makes one serving.

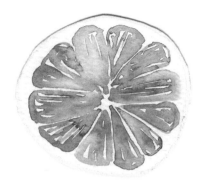

BOILERMAKER: WHEATGRASS

from Jason Harler and Tanya Hughes,
cofounders, American Medicinal Arts,
creators of holistic products and spa experiences

Get a cleansing energy boost: Knock back a shot of wheatgrass
and wash it down with fresh-squeezed citrus juice. The bright green
wheatgrass juice is also a potent killer of unwanted microorganisms.
Warrior food indeed! Here it makes sense to buy fresh wheatgrass
juice rather than the grass itself; juice the citrus yourself.

2 oranges, peeled; or 1 pink
   grapefruit, peeled
½ cup (40 ml) wheatgrass
   juice

Juice the wheatgrass and oranges separately. Serve the
wheatgrass shot with the citrus juice on the side.

Makes one serving.

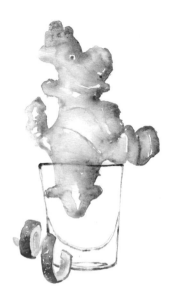

BOILERMAKER: GINGER
from Jason Harler and Tanya Hughes,
cofounders, American Medicinal Arts,
creators of holistic products and spa experiences

Get your internal digestive fire started with a shot of spicy ginger,
followed by a refreshing citrus chaser. Ginger also helps lower
inflammation and ease stomach upset.

3 inches (7 cm) fresh ginger
2 oranges, peeled; or 1 pink
  grapefruit, peeled

Juice the ginger and oranges separately. Serve the
ginger shot with the orange juice on the side.

Makes one serving.

· ·

GOOGLE SEASONAL
GINGER SHOT

from Rick Bender, chef, Google NY/
Restaurant Associates

Ginger has great anti-inflammatory benefits, and honey has great
antibacterial and antiviral properties. The heat and citrus in this shot also
fire up the digestive juices and jump-start detoxification. This powerfully
spicy shot is a great way to boost the immune system any time of year,
and is used as a base for the shots that follow.

· ·

1 inch (2.5 cm) fresh ginger
3 lemons, peeled
⅛ teaspoon ground cayenne
2 tablespoons raw honey

Juice the ginger and lemons, then stir in the cayenne
and honey and serve in a shot glass.

Makes one serving.

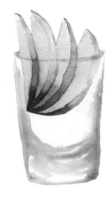

SPRING:
MANGO CURRY GINGER SHOT

Add some sweet, beta-carotene-rich mango
to the ginger and give your skin a nice antioxidant boost
to help protect it from the sun.

· ·

1 Google Seasonal Ginger
   Shot (page 73)
1½ tablespoons mango juice
Pinch curry powder

Stir all the ingredients together and serve
in a shot glass.

Makes one serving.

SUMMER:
STRAWBERRY RHUBARB GINGER SHOT

Sweet summer strawberries and sour rhubarb
complement the ginger for a refreshing flavor and
a boost of antioxidants.

· ·

1 Google Seasonal Ginger
   Shot (page 73)
1½ tablespoons strawberry
   juice
1 teaspoon rhubarb juice

Stir all the ingredients together
and serve in a shot glass.

Makes one serving.

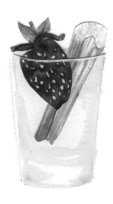

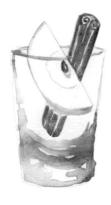

FALL:
MULLED APPLE GINGER SHOT

Warming spices and tart-sweet apple cider
make a comforting fall shot.

. . . .

1 Google Seasonal Ginger
   Shot (page 73)
1½ tablespoons apple cider
Pinch ground cinnamon
Pinch ground allspice

Stir all the ingredients together and serve
in a shot glass.

Makes one serving.

WINTER:
POMEGRANATE ORANGE GINGER SHOT

Oranges and pomegranates—two quintessential
winter fruits—offer plenty of antioxidants to help you
get through the colder months until spring's berries arrive,
and the ginger will warm you from the inside out.

. . . .

1 Google Seasonal Ginger
   Shot (page 73)
1 teaspoon pomegranate juice
1 teaspoon orange juice

Stir all the ingredients together
and serve in a shot glass.

Makes one serving.

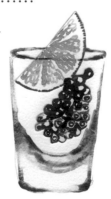

TART
+
CREAMY

Grapefruit + Orange + Lemon
Kale + Apple + Lemon
Parsley + Cucumber + Lemon
Peppers + Tomato
Pineapple + Lime + Cilantro
Romaine + Apple
Romaine + Celery + Lemon
Watercress + Pineapple
Tomato + Basil + Carrot

REFRESHING
+
LUSCIOUS

Beet + Apple
Carrot + Orange
Cucumber + Celery + Apple
Fennel + Cucumber + Lime
Greens + Pear + Grapefruit
Grapefruit + Kale + Apple
Kale + Pear + Cucumber
Orange + Greens
Pineapple + Kale
Pomegranate + Beet
Raspberry + Orange

COOLING
+
CRISP

Aloe + Lemon + Apple
Apple + Greens
Beet + Cucumber + Lime
Cucumber + Basil
Cucumber + Mint + Lime
Dandelion + Cucumber
Grapefruit + Mint
Greens + Mint + Pineapple
Greens + Cucumber + Mint
Grape + Fennel + Spinach
Watercress + Pear + Mint
Watermelon + Cucumber
Watermelon + Mint

RICH
+
TANGY

Cantaloupe + Nectarine
Grapefruit + Lime + Orange
Mango + Kale + Lime
Pear + Purslane

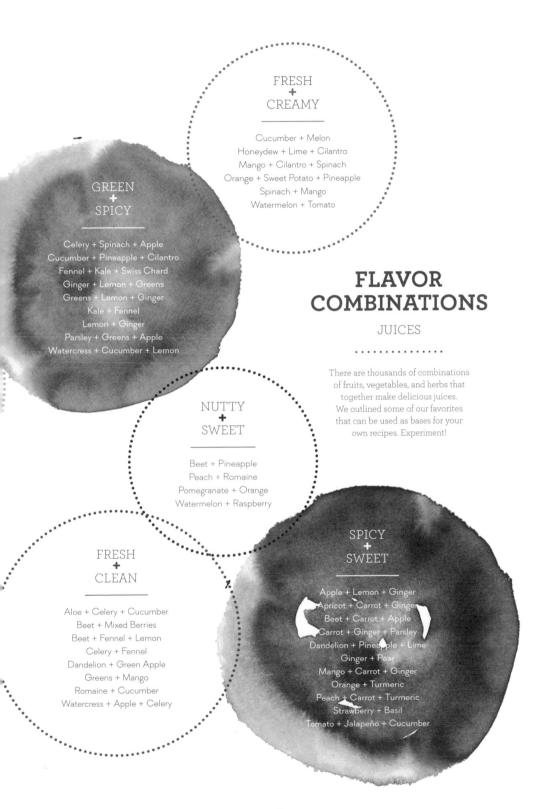

FRESH + CREAMY

Cucumber + Melon
Honeydew + Lime + Cilantro
Mango + Cilantro + Spinach
Orange + Sweet Potato + Pineapple
Spinach + Mango
Watermelon + Tomato

GREEN + SPICY

Celery + Spinach + Apple
Cucumber + Pineapple + Cilantro
Fennel + Kale + Swiss Chard
Ginger + Lemon + Greens
Greens + Lemon + Ginger
Kale + Fennel
Lemon + Ginger
Parsley + Greens + Apple
Watercress + Cucumber + Lemon

FLAVOR COMBINATIONS

JUICES

· · · · · · · · · · · ·

There are thousands of combinations
of fruits, vegetables, and herbs that
together make delicious juices.
We outlined some of our favorites
that can be used as bases for your
own recipes. Experiment!

NUTTY + SWEET

Beet + Pineapple
Peach + Romaine
Pomegranate + Orange
Watermelon + Raspberry

SPICY + SWEET

Apple + Lemon + Ginger
Apricot + Carrot + Ginger
Beet + Carrot + Apple
Carrot + Ginger + Parsley
Dandelion + Pineapple + Lime
Ginger + Pear
Mango + Carrot + Ginger
Orange + Turmeric
Peach + Carrot + Turmeric
Strawberry + Basil
Tomato + Jalapeño + Cucumber

FRESH + CLEAN

Aloe + Celery + Cucumber
Beet + Mixed Berries
Beet + Fennel + Lemon
Celery + Fennel
Dandelion + Green Apple
Greens + Mango
Romaine + Cucumber
Watercress + Apple + Celery

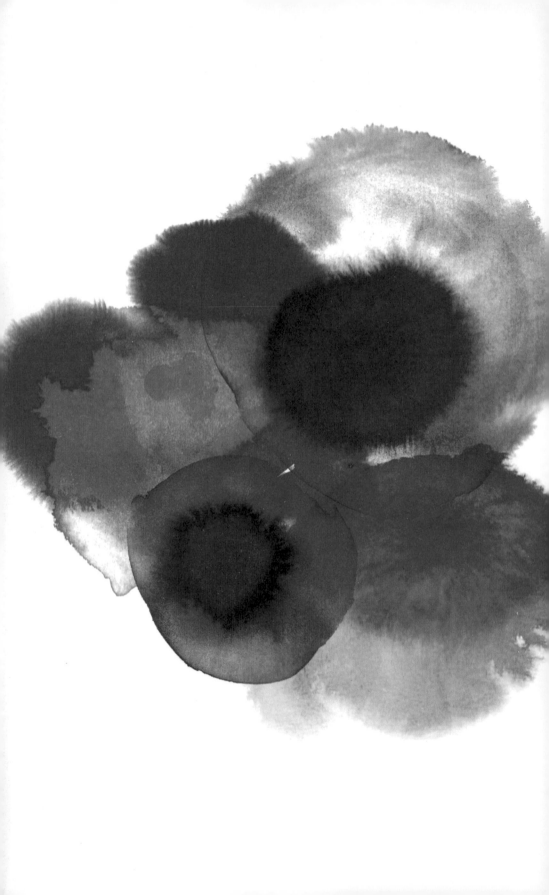

SMOOTHIES

The main difference between a smoothie and a juice is the pulp and fiber. In a juice, all the pulp has been removed and you're left with only liquid. A smoothie, on the other hand, consists of whole fruits or vegetables, usually with a base liquid and some-times with ice or other frozen ingredi-ents, blended into a thick liquid drink. The fiber remains in the drink, so you get all of its benefits: It's filling, so you stay satisfied for longer after you drink a smoothie; it helps slow down sugar absorption; and, of course, it helps keep you regular. Blending the fruits and vegetables makes their fiber easier to digest than if you were to just eat the ingredients on their own. Green smoothies—there are many wonderful ones in this chapter—are like shake versions of green juice, a drinkable salad of leafy greens, maybe some cucumber, celery, and apple, with a base that's often just filtered water or naturally sweet coconut water. If you're new to green smoothies, try adding a banana for a touch more sweetness and a bit of creaminess, and, if at all possible, use a good high-speed blender that can reduce those leafy greens to a pleasant, silky-smooth consistency. Toward the end of the chapter you'll find a collection of cold blended soups, which are basically savory smoothies that can be enjoyed as a meal in themselves (or as the opening act of an elegant multicourse dinner).

TIPS TO REMEMBER

- Always thoroughly wash fruits and vegetables prior to use.
- Core any apples or pears prior to use.
- Pit any stone fruits prior to use.
- Follow directions for your equipment. Centrifugal juicers can handle larger pieces of fruits and vegetables; masticating juicers and blenders require fruits and vegetables to be cut into smaller pieces.
- Volumes of final juices and smoothies can vary by more than 50 percent depending on the size of fruits and vegetables used and the type of juicer.
- Experiment! Once familiar with the recipes, try swapping in different berries, greens, or nut milks for different variations.
- If premaking smoothies, preblend any item with the exception of leafy greens and supplements. Add those items prior to serving.
- Serving sizes for supplements vary by brand. Follow instructions for suggested serving size.

MAKING NUT MILKS

There are several methods you can use to strain blended nuts
and water to make homemade nut milks. Perhaps the easiest
option is to pour the resulting slurry into a clean French press
coffee maker and depress the screen plunger to filter out
the fine nut solids.

Another method is to use a nut-milk bag: Pour the blended
mixture into the bag and squeeze all the liquid out into a bowl,
then discard the solids left in the bag.

You could also simply pour the blended mixture through a
very-fine-mesh sieve or several layers of rinsed and squeezed
cheesecloth into a bowl.

Note that for all of the following basic nondairy milk recipes,
dates, vanilla, and salt are optional.

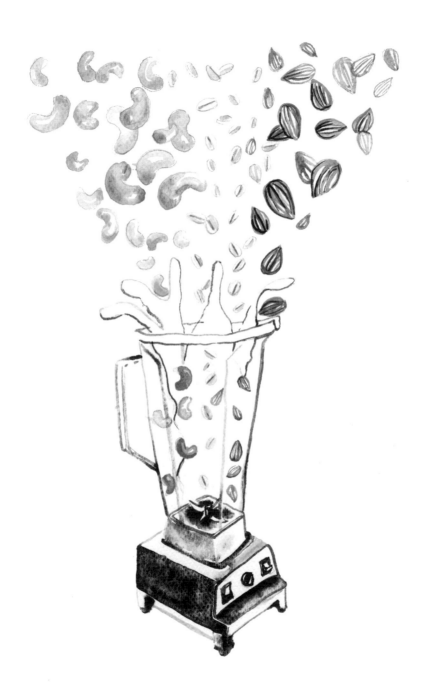

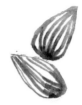

ALMOND NUT MILK
from The Juicery

No store-bought milk comes close to homemade almond milk—
not only is homemade more flavorful, with a more pleasing consistency,
but it also offers more nutritional benefits. It's a lot easier than you might
think to make nut milks at home. All you need is a blender and a French
press, a very-fine-mesh sieve, cheesecloth, or a nut-milk bag.

Almonds contain healthy fats, vitamin E, and calcium as well as protein.
Nut milks are a nutritious alternative to cow's milk for anyone who has
a dairy intolerance or simply prefers to avoid it.

1 cup (140 g) almonds,
soaked in water to cover
for at least 12 hours, then
drained and rinsed until
the water runs clear
2¾ cups (660 ml) filtered
water

Optional:
¼ teaspoon fine sea salt
1 teaspoon vanilla extract
2 Medjool dates, pitted

Blend the almonds, water, and salt, if using, in a high-
speed blender for 30 seconds. Strain the nut milk
using one of the methods described on page 82.
(If using vanilla and/or dates, return the strained liquid
to the blender, add the vanilla and dates, and blend
for 15 seconds, until smooth.) Serve, or store in a
covered container in the refrigerator for up to 3 days.

Makes four servings.

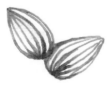

CASHEW NUT MILK

from Abigail James, international facialist
and well-being expert

Cashew nut milk is creamy and rich and packed with magnesium,
zinc, iron, and potassium—all of which are great for the skin.

1 cup (140 g) raw (unroasted) cashews, rinsed until the water runs clear, soaked in water to cover for at least 8 hours, then drained and rinsed until the water runs clear
3 cups (710 ml) filtered water
1⅓ cups (310 ml) unsweetened coconut water

Optional:
1 to 2 tablespoons maple syrup or raw honey
2 teaspoons vanilla extract
Pinch fine sea salt
Pinch ground cinnamon

Blend the cashews and 2 cups (470 ml) of the filtered water until very smooth, starting on low speed and increasing the speed to high; this could take 2 or more minutes. Add the remaining 1 cup (240 ml) water, the coconut water, and maple syrup, vanilla, salt, and cinnamon, if using, and blend until smooth. If your blender can't break down the cashews completely, strain the nut milk using one of the methods described on page 82. Cover and refrigerate for up to 4 days.

Makes five servings.

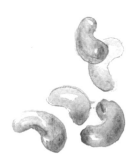

PISTACHIO NUT MILK

from Julie Elliott, founder, In Fiore

Love pistachio ice cream? Then you're going to love this
guilt-free unsweetened nut milk version. Pistachios are actually lower
in fats and calories than other nuts, yet packed with flavor.

1 cup (130 g) unsalted shelled pistachios, rinsed until the water runs clear, soaked in water to cover for 5 hours, then drained and rinsed until the water runs clear

1 quart (1 liter) filtered water, plus more if desired.

Rub off the pistachio skins. Put the pistachios and water in a blender and blend until smooth, adding more water to achieve the texture you want. Cover and refrigerate for up to 4 days.

Makes four servings.

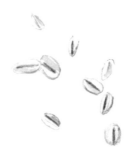

OAT MILK
from Les Fermes de Marie

Mild and light oat milk makes an excellent substitute for dairy or nut milk.

1 cup (80 g) rolled oats
2 cups (470 ml) filtered water

Optional:
Pinch fine sea salt

In a large bowl, combine the oats and water; cover and let soak overnight. Transfer to a blender and blend until very smooth, about 2 minutes. Strain the oat milk using one of the methods described on page 82. Stir in the salt, if using. Cover and refrigerate for up to 3 days.

Makes two servings.

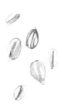

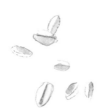

COCONUT MILK
The Juicery

To extract more fat from the coconut, bring the water to a simmer
and pour it over the coconut in the blender. Let the mixture cool
to room temperature for approximately 30 minutes before blending—
just be sure to vent the blender lid and put a towel over the top
to prevent explosions. Let cool to room temperature before adding
the vanilla and dates or honey.

2 cups (180 g) shredded,
  unsweetened coconut
4 cups (880 ml) filtered water
  (reduce to 2 cups [440 ml]
  for a richer milk)

Optional:
Pinch fine sea salt
1 teaspoon vanilla extract,
  or the seeds of 1 vanilla bean
  (see Note)
2 Medjool dates, pitted,
  or raw honey

Blend the coconut, water, and salt, if using, until very
smooth, starting on low speed and increasing the
speed to high; this could take 2 or more minutes. If
your blender can't break down the coconut completely,
strain the coconut milk using one of the methods
described on page 82. Stir in the vanilla and blend in
the dates or honey, if using. Cover and refrigerate for
up to 4 days in a bottle. The coconut milk will separate
in the refrigerator into a layer of thick coconut oil on
the top and water on the bottom; before using, gently
warm it by putting the bottle in a pan of hot water for
a few minutes, then shaking it to disperse the oil.

Makes four servings.

Note: To use a vanilla bean, split it lengthwise in half with a sharp
knife and scrape the seeds from the inside; use the seeds in the
recipe, and save the vanilla bean pod to use for infusing hot drinks.

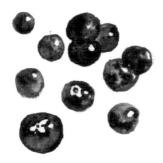

DR. JUNGER'S MORNING SMOOTHIE

from Dr. Alejandro Junger, medical director and creator,
the Clean Program

Why not enjoy a rich chocolate smoothie first thing in the morning?
Almonds provide healthy fats, protein, and fiber, and blueberries and
unsweetened cocoa are high in antioxidants. Cacao also serves as an energy
booster, making this smoothie the perfect start to the morning.

¼ avocado
1⅓ cups (320 ml) almond
 nut milk, preferably
 homemade (page 84)
1 teaspoon unsweetened
 cocoa powder
⅔ cup (100 g) blueberries
1 teaspoon almond butter
2 ice cubes

Recommended supplement:
1½ teaspoons pea protein

Blend all the ingredients together. Serve immediately.

Makes one serving.

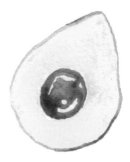

··

COMO MUSCLE THERAPY
from Eve Persak, M.S., R.D., C.N.S.C.,
and Amanda Gale, COMO Shambhala

Subtly spiced with cinnamon and cacao nibs, and enriched with
coconut meat, this naturally sweet smoothie speeds recovery by reducing
inflammation and replenishing electrolytes and nutrients.

··

1 banana
1 cup (240 g) ice cubes made
  with unsweetened coconut
  water
1½ cups (350 ml) almond nut
  milk, preferably homemade
  (page 84)
½ cup (40 g) fresh or frozen
  coconut meat
Pinch ground cinnamon
1 tablespoon ground flaxseeds
4 Medjool dates, pitted and
  minced
1 teaspoon cacao nibs,
  ground, or unsweetened
  cocoa powder

Blend all the ingredients together. Serve immediately.

Makes one serving.

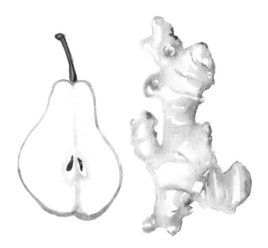

DR. LIPMAN'S
GINGER PEAR SMOOTHIE
from Dr. Frank Lipman, founder and director,
Eleven Eleven Wellness Center & Be Well

This sweet-tart shake has great anti-inflammatory properties, and the pear is cooling. Pear and ginger also both help soothe a sore throat.

1½ pears, cored
¾ cup (180 ml) almond nut milk, preferably homemade (page 84)
1¼ inches (3 cm) fresh ginger, peeled
4 teaspoons fresh lime juice
2 teaspoons vanilla extract
4 ice cubes

Recommended supplement:
2 teaspoons greens powder, preferably Be Well Super-greens Powder

Blend all the ingredients together. Serve immediately. If not serving immediately, blend all but the ice and greens powder and refrigerate, then blend in the ice and greens powder just before serving.

Makes one serving.

PEANUT BUTTER CHOCOLATE SHAKE
The Juicery

Protein is essential for muscle recovery after a tough workout, and the peanuts and pea protein in this subtly sweet shake provide lots—and all from plant sources. Cacao is a powerful antioxidant that helps fight stress and gives you a little extra energy boost after all that hard work. Banana provides potassium that helps fight off muscle cramping.

. . . .

1 cup (240 ml) almond nut
   milk, preferably homemade
   (page 84), or water
½ banana
1 tablespoon peanut butter
1½ tablespoons raw cacao
   powder
3 ice cubes

Recommended supplement:
1 serving pea protein

Blend all the ingredients together. Serve immediately.

Makes one serving.

A.J.'S POWER SMOOTHIE
from Kris Carr, author, with Chad Sarno,
Crazy Sexy Kitchen

Fortified with both nut milk and almond butter and slightly sweetened with fruit you could pull straight from the freezer, this light green smoothie would make an easy everyday drink. The quality of your cinnamon will make all the difference here: Look for dark-hued Vietnamese cinnamon, which when fresh can taste almost sweet!

. . . .

3 cups nut milk (710 ml)
   preferably homemade
   (pages 84–86)
½ cup (30 g) fresh or frozen
   berries
½ cup (40 g) frozen mango
5 kale leaves
Handful spinach
2 tablespoons raw almond
   butter
Pinch ground cinnamon

Blend all the ingredients together. Serve immediately, blended with ice, poured over ice cubes, or at room temperature with no ice.

Makes one serving.

SPICY CHAI MILK
The Juicery

Warming and sweet spices make this drink a great winter treat. Drink it chilled or heat it up for a relaxing, soothing, and comforting cup.

2 cups (470 ml) almond nut
   milk (use less if adding ice),
   preferably homemade
   (page 84)
1 large Medjool date,
   or 4 small dates, pitted
½ teaspoon vanilla extract,
   or the seeds of 1 vanilla
   bean (see Note, page 88)
½ teaspoon ground cinnamon
Pinch ground cardamom
Pinch fine sea salt

Optional:
5 ice cubes

Recommended supplement:
1 heaping teaspoon mixed
   greens powder

Blend all the ingredients together. Serve cold, or omit the ice cubes and warm the mixture in a small saucepan until steaming and serve hot.

Makes one serving.

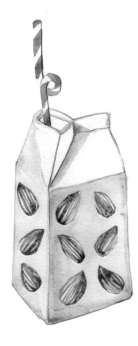

93

CHOCOLATE MINT MILK
The Juicery

Better than any chocolate milk you've ever had,
this is a real grown-up version with just the right balance
of sweet, cool, bitter, and creamy.

2 cups (470 ml) almond nut
milk (use less if adding ice),
preferably homemade
(page 84)
1 large Medjool date
or 4 small dates, pitted
6 mint leaves
1½ tablespoons raw cacao
powder
1 teaspoon cacao nibs
Pinch sea salt

Optional:
5 ice cubes

Recommended supplement:
½ teaspoon maca

Blend all the ingredients together. Serve immediately.

Makes one serving.

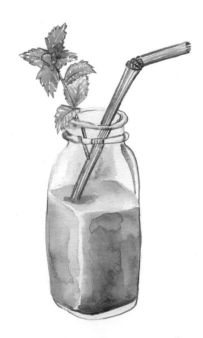

MELROSE SMOOTHIE
The Juicery

The mango in this sweet-tart smoothie is great for your skin
and contains plenty of vitamin C for immunity.

· ·

1 cup (240 ml) almond nut
  milk, preferably homemade
  (page 84)
½ banana
1½ cups (250 g) mango
3 ice cubes

Blend all the ingredients together. Serve immediately.

Makes one serving.

FOUNTAIN SMOOTHIE
The Juicery

This drink—tart and fresh-tasting—is a serious skin elixir,
with both beta-carotene from mango and a high dose of vitamin C
from the bright orange sea buckthorn berries. Vitamin C is an
antioxidant that helps repair and regenerate collagen, and collagen
is what keeps your skin plump and youthful.

· ·

¼ cup (40 g) sea buckthorn
  berries, fresh or frozen
1 cup (170 g) mango
1 cup (240 ml) almond nut
  milk, preferably homemade
  (page 84)
4 ice cubes

Optional:
1 teaspoon raw honey

Juice the berries and mango. Stir in the almond milk
and honey, if using. Blend with ice. Serve immediately.

Makes one serving.

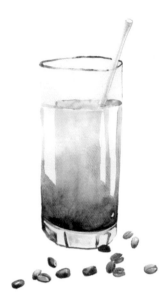

BLACK AND TAN
The Juicery

Rise and shine with a whole new take on coffee. The Black and Tan is creamy
and bittersweet, with a touch of cinnamon and chia for good measure.
Blackstrap molasses is great for boosting iron levels.

1 cup plus 2 tablespoons
   nut milk (280 ml) such as
   almond, preferably homemade (page 84), or hemp
2 shots (170 ml) brewed
   espresso
1 tablespoon blackstrap
   molasses
½ teaspoon ground cinnamon
1 tablespoon chia seeds

Blend all the ingredients together, adding more nut
milk for a less-intense drink. Serve immediately.

Makes one serving.

SEXY SUPERFOOD SMOOTHIE

from Saimaa Miller, naturopath and author,
Aussie Body Diet and Detox Plan, Aussie Body Diet Pty. Ltd.

Think of this as the most nutritious, healthful chocolate shake
you could ask for: lightly sweetened with frozen banana and maple syrup,
flavored with deep, dark raw cacao and pure vanilla.

1½ cups (350 ml) almond nut
  milk, preferably homemade
  (page 84)
1 small banana, chopped
  and frozen
1 tablespoon maca powder
1 tablespoon raw cacao powder
1 tablespoon flaxseed oil
1 teaspoon maple syrup
½ teaspoon vanilla extract
Pinch Celtic sea salt
  or Himalayan salt

Recommended supplement:
1 tablespoon hemp protein
  powder

Blend all the ingredients together. Serve immediately.

Makes one serving.

VANILLA
GREEN TEA SMOOTHIE

from Jennifer Maanavi and Tanya Becker, cofounders, Physique 57

A super-simple and easy-to-make post-workout smoothie,
this green tea latte is loaded with antioxidants and healthy fats.

. . . .

1½ cups (350 ml) almond nut
milk, preferably homemade
(page 84)
1 teaspoon vanilla
extract
½ teaspoon powdered green
tea (also known as matcha
powder)
1 tablespoon grade-B
maple syrup
5 ice cubes

Optional:
Pinch fine sea salt

Blend all the ingredients together. Serve immediately.

Makes one serving.

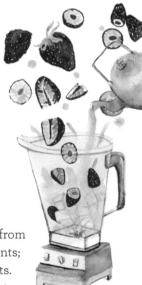

STRAWBERRY
GREEN TEA SMOOTHIE

from Nini Ordoubadi, founder, Tay Tea

This shake contains matcha, a finely ground powder from
young green tea leaves that is loaded with antioxidants;
look for it in natural foods stores and Asian markets.
It also contains a little caffeine, making this a great
shake when you need a boost of energy.

. . . .

¾ cup (180 ml) almond nut
milk, preferably homemade
(page 84)
¼ cup (60 ml) filtered water
1 cup (144 g) strawberries
1½ teaspoons matcha
(green tea) powder
5 ice cubes

Blend all the ingredients together. Serve immediately.

Makes one serving.

BANANA BLUEBERRY OAT SMOOTHIE
from Cal-a-Vie

This is a great, filling, rich, and satisfying breakfast
alternative packed with fiber, protein, and healthy fats:
a complete meal in a glass!

1 large frozen banana
½ cup (80 g) fresh or frozen
   blueberries
¼ cup (20 g) rolled oats
1 tablespoon ground flaxseed
1 cup (240 ml) almond nut
   milk, preferably homemade
   (page 84)
⅛ teaspoon ground cinnamon

Recommended supplement:
1 tablespoon whey protein
   powder

Blend all the ingredients together. Serve immediately.

Makes one serving.

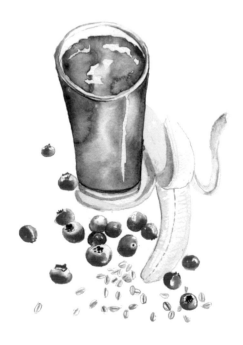

KALE MINT
LEMONGRASS SMOOTHIE

from Dr. Amy Myers, M.D. and author

This cool, herbal, lemongrass-scented smoothie, sweetened
and thickened a bit with frozen banana and given a nutrient boost
with tender, mineral-rich baby kale, is worth making even if you don't
choose to add the supplements.

1 cup (240 ml) almond nut
  milk, preferably homemade
  (page 84)
1 frozen banana
Very large handful baby kale
6 mint leaves
1 inch (2.5 cm) lemongrass,
  finely chopped
6 ice cubes

Recommended supplements:
1 serving L-glutamine powder
¼ teaspoon probiotic powder
¼ teaspoon immune booster

Blend all the ingredients together. Serve immediately.

Makes one serving.

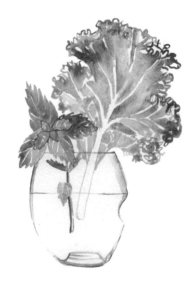

STONE FRUIT SMOOTHIE

from Alex Glasscock, founder and owner, The Ranch at Live Oak, Malibu

The apricot and peach season is short, but oh so sweet.
Packed with vitamins B and C plus a load of beta-carotene,
here the summery fruits are blended with creamy almond milk
and sweet and sour raspberries. Refresh, recharge, and rejoice!

· ·

½ cup (120 ml) almond nut
   milk, preferably homemade
   (page 84)
2 peaches, pitted
1 apricot, pitted
1 cup (120 g) frozen raspberries
2 tablespoons flaxseeds
4 ice cubes

Recommended supplement:
1 serving supergreens powder

Blend all the ingredients together. Serve immediately.

Makes one serving.

VA-VA VOOM

from the Herb House at Limewood

Just a touch of fragrant lavender ups the sophistication level
of this creamy, sweet periwinkle-colored smoothie.

· ·

1⅓ cups (320 ml) almond nut
   milk, preferably homemade
   (page 84) or rice milk
Handful blueberries
Tiny pinch dried lavender
   buds
2 teaspoons raw honey
¼ teaspoon vanilla extract

Blend all the ingredients together. Serve immediately,
blended with ice, poured over ice cubes, or at room
temperature with no ice.

Makes one serving.

COOL CUCUMBER LIME SMOOTHIE
from Alex Glasscock, founder and owner,
The Ranch at Live Oak, Malibu

. . . .

⅓ cup (80 ml) almond nut
  milk, preferably homemade
  (page 84)
12 inches (30 cm) cucumber,
  peeled and seeded
10 frozen green grapes
1 tablespoon fresh lime juice
½ teaspoon chopped mint
  leaves
4 ice cubes

Recommended supplement:
1 serving supergreens powder

Blend all the ingredients together. Serve immediately.

Makes one serving.

AB&J SMOOTHIE
from Alex Glasscock, founder and owner, The Ranch at Live Oak, Malibu

A creamy, sweet, and delicious treat with a nod to childhood's
peanut butter and jelly sandwiches, but made with nutritious
almond butter and raspberries instead.

. . . .

½ cup (120 ml) almond nut
  milk, preferably homemade
  (page 84)
2 cups (250 g) frozen
  raspberries
1 frozen banana
2 teaspoons almond butter
4 ice cubes

Recommended supplement:
1 serving supergreens powder

Blend all the ingredients together. Serve immediately.

Makes one serving.

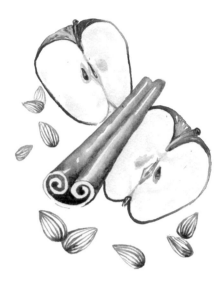

APPLE PIE SMOOTHIE

from Alex Glasscock, founder and owner,
The Ranch at Live Oak, Malibu

Sweet and homey as apple pie, but bursting with
micronutrients and healthy fats from the almonds, this is
a dessert you can feel good about.

⅔ cup (160 ml) almond nut
milk, preferably homemade
(page 84)
1 frozen banana
1 red apple, cored and
chopped
5 raw almonds
2 teaspoons almond butter
½ teaspoon ground cinnamon

Recommended supplement:
1 serving supergreens powder

Blend all the ingredients together. Serve immediately.

Makes one serving.

MINT HEMP-SEED SMOOTHIE

The Juicery

A refreshing and cooling smoothie with hemp seeds
for added protein and healthy fats.

1 frozen banana
1 tablespoon hemp seeds
Juice of ½ lime
8 to 10 mint leaves
1⅓ cups (320 ml) almond nut
  milk, preferably homemade
  (page 84)

Recommended supplement:
1 teaspoon barley grass powder

Blend all the ingredients together. Serve immediately.

Makes one serving.

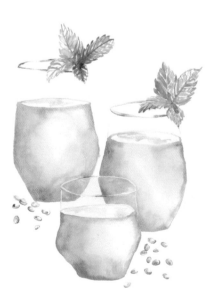

ESPRESSO MACA
The Juicery

A creamy and frothy coffee milkshake that will make you forget
about diner coffee and fast-food milkshakes once and for all.
The added maca gives the drink a subtle butterscotch flavor and has
great energizing and hormone-balancing benefits.

· ·

1 cup (240 ml) almond nut
  milk, preferably homemade
  (page 84)
¼ cup (60 ml) brewed
  espresso, cooled
2 Medjool dates, pitted
1 teaspoon almond butter
1 tablespoon maca powder
6 ice cubes

Blend all the ingredients together. Serve immediately.

Makes one serving.

ESPRESSO GINGER
The Juicery

This coffee drink turns up the heat with cinnamon and ginger.
Ginger has great anti-inflammatory benefits, and cinnamon
has been shown to help stabilize blood sugar. As an added bonus,
rooibos tea is packed with antioxidants!

· ·

¾ cup (180 ml) almond nut
  milk, preferably homemade
  (page 84)
½ cup (120 ml) brewed
  espresso, cooled
1 to 2 Medjool dates, pitted
2 tablespoons minced fresh
  ginger
½ teaspoon rooibos tea leaves
½ teaspoon ground cinnamon
6 ice cubes

Blend all the ingredients together. Serve immediately.

Makes one serving.

· ·

CHOCOLATE ESPRESSO SMOOTHIE

from David Laris, founder, David Laris Creates

Bulked up with antioxidant-containing beets and sweetened
with just a bit of honey if you like, this deep dark chocolate smoothie
would make an excellent afternoon pick-me-up. If the chocolate
doesn't do it, the shot of espresso will.

· ·

½ cup (150 g) beets
1⅓ cups (320 ml) almond nut
 milk, preferably homemade
 (page 84)
2 tablespoons brewed
 espresso, cooled
1 tablespoon raw cacao
 powder

Optional:
4 teaspoons raw honey

Juice the beets. Transfer to a blender, add the
remaining ingredients, and blend until smooth. Serve
immediately, blended with ice, poured over ice cubes,
or at room temperature with no ice.

Makes one serving.

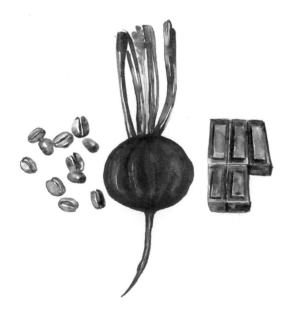

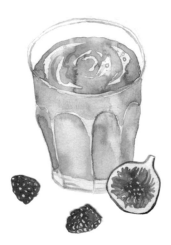

ROOIBOS CHIA SMOOTHIE
The Juicery

Rooibos is a surprising, nutritious, and delicious base for a smoothie,
packed with minerals and antioxidants. The chia seeds provide
filling fiber and those essential omega-3 fatty acids that so many of us
just don't get enough of. Fresh figs are sweet but also loaded with fiber.
Goji berries are great for energy and boosting your mood. Along with
the beet, they give this smoothie its beautiful pink color.

1 small beet
½ cup (120 ml) almond nut
  milk, preferably homemade
  (page 84)
½ cup (120 ml) chilled rooibos
  tea
2 fresh figs
1 Medjool date, pitted
2 tablespoons goji berries
  or goji berry powder
1 tablespoon chia seeds
½ cup (60 g) raspberries
½ teaspoon ground cinnamon,
  plus more for garnish
4 ice cubes

Juice the beet. Transfer to a blender, add the
remaining ingredients, and blend until smooth. Serve
immediately, garnished with a sprinkle of cinnamon.

Makes one serving.

· ·

APRICOT WITH PISTACHIO MILK, HONEY, AND ROSE SMOOTHIE

from Julie Elliott, founder, In Fiore

This subtly sweet drink is rich in vitamin C, which is what boosts collagen production, keeping our skin looking plump, elastic, and youthful. Apricots strengthen the immune system and have more carotene than any other fruit.

· ·

3 ripe apricots, pitted
½ cup (120 ml) pistachio nut
  milk, preferably homemade
  (page 86)
½ cup (120 ml) plain yogurt
1 tablespoon raw honey
1 tablespoon walnut butter,
  or other nut butter
1 tablespoon flaxseed oil
1 teaspoon royal jelly

Recommended supplements:
½ teaspoon rose hydrolate
1 serving probiotics

Blend all the ingredients together. Serve immediately.

Makes one serving.

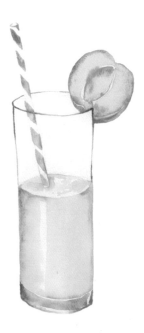

· ·

CHOCOLATE SURPRISE SMOOTHIE
from Dr. Frank Lipman, founder and director,
Eleven Eleven Wellness Center & Be Well

Here tangy but sweet blueberries (try to find the tiny wild ones,
fresh or frozen; they have more flavor than cultivated varieties) and chocolate
whey powder complement the smoothie's creamy elements.

· ·

1 cup (220 ml) unsweetened
  almond nut milk or
  coconut milk, preferably
  homemade (pages 84, 88),
  or half water and half
  coconut milk
¼ avocado
1 cup (50 g) tightly packed
  kale
1 cup (150 g) blueberries
1 tablespoon chia seeds
5 ice cubes

Recommended supplements:
1 serving Be Well chocolate
  whey powder
1 serving Be Well Phyto
  Greens powder

Blend all the ingredients together. Serve immediately.

Makes one serving.

SNOW VELVET SMOOTHIE
from Les Fermes de Marie

Cozy up to the fire with this yummy wintry treat. With its warming spices, creamy oat milk, and fiber-rich, sweet fruits, who needs cookies?

. . . .

4 apples
2 pears
1 cup (240 ml) oat milk, preferably homemade (page 87)
½ teaspoon gingerbread powder or substitute with a pumpkin pie spice mix

Juice the apples and pears. Transfer to a blender and blend with the oat milk and gingerbread powder. Serve immediately, blended with ice, poured over ice cubes, or at room temperature with no ice.

Makes one serving.

CRAZY CACAO SMOOTHIE
from Saimaa Miller, naturopath and author,
Aussie Body Diet and Detox Plan, Aussie Body Diet Pty. Ltd.

Dates and raw cacao are a match made in heaven. You can, of course, use any kind of milk you'd like here, but the strong flavors of cinnamon and chocolate take especially well to nutty brown rice milk.

. . . .

2 cups (470 ml) brown rice milk
1 small banana, chopped and frozen
1 Medjool date, pitted and soaked in water to cover until soft
2 tablespoons raw cacao powder
2 tablespoons hemp seed oil
½ teaspoon ground cinnamon
Ice cubes

Blend all the ingredients together. Serve immediately.

Makes one serving.

BRAIN-BOOSTING TONIC

from Kara Rosen, founder, Plenish Cleanse

We could all use a little help with our memory, especially as we age.
Why not get help in the form of a delicious, milky green smoothie?
Chia seeds are high in omega-3 fatty acids, which support memory function.
Bonus: The calcium and magnesium in the greens here strengthen
bones and fight menopausal symptoms.

½ cup (50 g) tightly packed
spinach
½ cup (50 g) tightly packed
watercress
1½ cups (350 ml) almond or
cashew nut milk, preferably
homemade (pages 84, 85)
½ cup (70 g) frozen or fresh
blueberries
4 to 5 sprigs parsley
1 teaspoon maca powder
1 teaspoon chia seeds

Juice the spinach and watercress. Transfer to a
blender, add the remaining ingredients, and blend until
smooth. (Alternatively, skip the juicing and blend
the spinach and watercress along with the rest of the
ingredients.) Serve immediately, blended with ice,
poured over ice cubes, or at room temperature with
no ice.

Makes one serving.

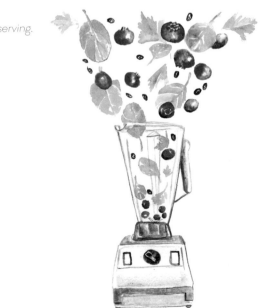

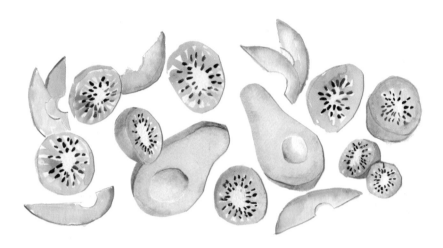

DR. LIPMAN'S KIWI AVOCADO SHAKE

from Dr. Frank Lipman, founder and director,
Eleven Eleven Wellness Center & Be Well

Kiwi is high in vitamin C and low in sugar. Greens and fats are great
for the skin, and with protein added, this tart, creamy smoothie is good
for post-workout replenishment.

1 cup (40 g) spinach
½ cup (120 ml) unsweetened
  coconut milk
½ cup (120 ml) filtered water
2 kiwis, peeled
¼ avocado
4 ice cubes

Recommended supplement:
1 tablespoon pea protein

Blend all the ingredients together. Serve immediately.

Makes one serving.

DOCTOR-DESIGNED ANTI-INFLAMMATORY AND GUT-HEALING SMOOTHIE

from Dr. Amy Myers, M.D. and author

Nearly every ingredient in this sweet-spiced tropical smoothie has anti-inflammatory and gut-healing properties. Mangos are rich in antioxidants, vitamins A and C, and immunity-boosting carotenoids; papayas contain protein-digesting enzymes that help reduce inflammation; the gingerol in ginger is an anti-inflammatory; turmeric contains the antioxidant, anti-inflammatory compound called curcumin; cinnamon reduces inflammatory regulatory molecules in the body; and flaxseeds, chia seeds, and walnuts are rich in omega-3s, which are potent anti-inflammatory aids.

1½ cups (350 ml) unsweetened flaxseed milk
½ cup (80 g) chopped frozen mango
½ cup (80 g) papaya
¼ cup (40 g) walnuts, finely ground if not using a high-speed blender
½ inch fresh ginger
½ inch fresh turmeric root
½ teaspoon ground cinnamon
1 tablespoon chia seeds, finely ground if not using a high-speed blender
1 tablespoon flaxseeds, finely ground if not using a high-speed blender

Recommended supplements:
1 serving L-glutamine powder
¼ teaspoon probiotic powder

Blend all the ingredients together. Serve immediately.

Makes one serving.

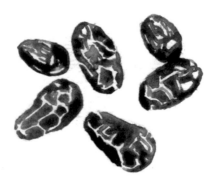

CARDAMOM COCONUT DATE SMOOTHIE
The Juicery

This drink is packed with healthy fats and sweetened with luscious dates. Warm spices and a nutty almond-butter component make it soothing and comforting for the soul. And cinnamon even helps balance blood-sugar levels.

2 large Medjool dates,
   or 4 small dates, pitted
1 tablespoon almond butter
1 cup (240 ml) unsweetened
   coconut milk, preferably
   homemade (page 88)
2 teaspoons shredded,
   unsweetened coconut
4 ice cubes
Pinch ground cinnamon

Blend the dates, almond butter, coconut milk, coconut, and ice together. Serve immediately, garnished with the cinnamon.

Makes one serving.

POST-YOGA SMOOTHIE

from Tiffany Cruikshank, Pure Yoga, New York

This green smoothie gives you a nice boost of energy following a workout.
The good fats from the avocado will help you feel more satiated
and balance blood sugar for a more even mood. The greens replenish
the muscles with magnesium, and the cantaloupe and coconut water
are packed with potassium; magnesium and potassium enhance muscle
functioning by allowing the muscles to contract to their full potential
and to relax and avoid cramping. Spinach is loaded with iron and helps carry
oxygen through the body (citric acid in the lemon juice helps
the body absorb the iron in the spinach). Matcha contains caffeine,
but it's also loaded with valuable antioxidants.

¼ avocado
½ to 1 cup (80 to 160 g)
   cantaloupe
Handful spinach
1 to 2 kale, chard, or collard
   green leaves, tough stems
   and ribs removed
Small squeeze of fresh lemon
   juice
1 cup (240 ml) unsweetened
   coconut water
Filtered water as needed

Optional:
1 teaspoon matcha
   (green tea) powder
5 to 6 basil leaves
4 ice cubes

Recommended supplement:
1 serving pure whey protein,
   or 2 tablespoons hemp seeds

Blend all the ingredients together, adding water as
needed to achieve the desired consistency. Serve
immediately, blended with ice, poured over ice cubes,
or at room temperature with no ice.

Makes one serving.

. . . .

CRAZY SEXY
GODDESS SMOOTHIE

from Kris Carr, author, and Chad Sarno, chef,
Crazy Sexy Kitchen

The avocado in this sweet smoothie provides not only healthy fats
but also dairy-free creaminess and body.

. . . .

1 avocado
1 banana
1 cup (150 g) blueberries
12 inches (30 cm) cucumber
Handful kale, romaine, lettuce,
  or spinach
½ cup (120 ml) unsweetened
  coconut water or filtered
  water, as needed

Optional:
Stevia and/or ground cinnamon
  or ground cacao nibs to taste

Recommended supplements:
1 to 2 tablespoons E3 Live

Blend all the ingredients together, adding coconut
water or filtered water as needed to achieve the
desired consistency. Serve immediately, blended
with ice, poured over ice cubes, or at room temperature
with no ice.

Makes one serving.

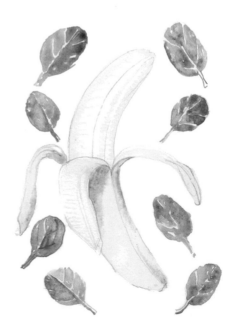

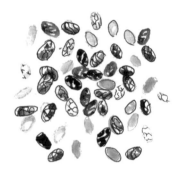

SWEET 'N' SMOOTH BREAKFAST SMOOTHIE

from Marcelle Pick, R.N.C., M.S.N., OB/GYN NP,
best-selling author and cofounder, Women to Women

Super-simple, sweet, and tart, this is one smoothie you'll want to
turn to often when mangos are ripe and in season—early summer in most
areas. Consider buying lots of the fruit when they're inexpensive
and at their best, and freezing them for use later.

1½ cups (350 ml) unsweet-
  ened coconut water or
  filtered water
1 mango, peeled
2 handfuls spinach
1 heaping tablespoon chia
  seeds

Recommended supplement:
1 serving gluten-free, sugar-
  free protein powder

Blend all the ingredients together, adding coconut
water as needed to achieve the desired consistency.
Serve immediately, blended with ice, poured over
ice cubes, or at room temperature with no ice.

Makes one serving.

CREAMSICLE SMOOTHIE
The Juicery

This is a deliciously rich and creamy shake packed with nutrients
and without any of the guilt associated with its namesake novelty
ice cream treat. If you're up for a really cooling experience, pour the
citrusy mixture into ice pop molds and enjoy it frozen!

. . . .

½ cup (90 g) frozen mango
½ cup (120 ml) unsweetened
  coconut water
½ cup (120 ml) unsweetened
  coconut milk, preferably
  homemade (page 88)
½ orange, peeled
4 ice cubes

Blend all the ingredients together. Serve immediately.

Makes one serving.

VINA-COLADA
The Juicery

This tropical delight is loaded with electrolytes, healthy fats,
and protein, perfect after a workout or for breakfast. (Or, really, any time
you feel like an imaginary escape to a warm, sunny island.)

. . . .

¾ cup (180 ml) unsweetened
  coconut water
½ tablespoon shredded,
  unsweetened coconut
½ serving vanilla whey
  powder
1 long slice mango
½ banana
¼ lime, peeled

Blend all the ingredients together. Serve immediately.

Makes one serving.

ENERGY BOOSTER SMOOTHIE

from Michelle Roques-O'Neil, aromatherapist, healer,
spiritual life coach, and natural perfumer

This is an all-in-one kick-start of a smoothie. Packed with antioxidants,
omega-3s, vitamins, and minerals, it's also delicious enough
to be a daily routine: nutty and sweet, with a hint of berry-tart freshness.
CoQ10 is an antioxidant that the body produces, though often not
enough of, leading to a lack of energy and general fatigue.
Adding some to your smoothie will help increase your energy levels
by allowing cells to function as efficiently as possible.

1 cup (240 ml) unsweetened
  coconut water
⅓ cup (80 ml) almond nut
  milk, preferably homemade
  (page 84)
½ banana
½ pear
Handful raspberries
Raw honey to taste

Recommended supplements:
1 tablespoon Linwoods milled
  flaxseed, goji berry, Brazil
  nut, or CoQ10 mix
½ teaspoon wheatgrass
  powder
½ teaspoon baobab powder
½ teaspoon maca powder

Blend all the ingredients together. Serve immediately.

Makes one serving.

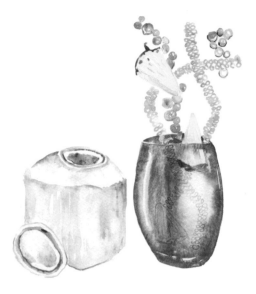

OCEAN SMOOTHIE
The Juicery

Here's a simple, slightly sweet smoothie that's refreshing, hydrating, and cooling on a hot summer day or just after a sweaty workout.

2½ inches (6 cm) cucumber
¾ cup (120 g) pineapple
½ cup (120 ml) unsweetened
   coconut water
2 ice cubes
1 teaspoon sea vegetable
   powder

Juice the cucumber and pineapple, then transfer to a blender, add the remaining ingredients, and blend until smooth. Serve immediately.

Makes one serving.

DR. JUNGER'S MALTED MILKSHAKE

from Dr. Alejandro Junger, medical director and creator,
the Clean Program

This is a real favorite among the Juicery's guests, and for good reason.
It's sweet, vicious, and totally delicious! Full of filling fiber and
a caramely richness from the dates, this tastes much more like a treat
than a health drink. Good thing is—it's both.

. . . .

2 cups (470 ml) unsweetened
  coconut water
1 tablespoon almond butter
5 Medjool dates, pitted
6 ice cubes

Recommended supplement:
1 serving whey or pea protein
  powder

Blend all the ingredients together. Serve immediately.
If not serving immediately, blend all but the ice and
protein powder, then blend in the protein powder and
ice just before serving.

Makes one serving.

WELL+GOOD MORNING TONIC

from Melisse Gelula and Alexia Brue, cofounders, Well+Good

Start your morning off right with this citrusy, light green
alkalizing tonic to help hydrate, soothe, and cleanse. Dandelion root
tea is a powerful detox booster and great for aiding digestion
and weight loss. Aloe vera has great digestive benefits and is soothing
for the skin. This drink is very low in sugar, which helps to maintain
stable blood-sugar levels and stave off cravings.

. . . .

½ cup (120 ml) coconut water
½ cup (120 ml) brewed
  dandelion root tea, chilled
1 teaspoon aloe vera juice
1 cup (40 g) kale, or 1 serving
  organic greens powder
¼ lemon, with peel
½ green apple

Optional:
½ frozen banana or
  ½ avocado
1 serving of any herbal tincture
  (available at most health
  food stores)

Blend all ingredients and serve immediately.
Adding the banana or avocado turns this into
a pre-workout smoothie.

Makes one serving.

· ·

CREAMY COCONUT
MACA SMOOTHIE
from Saimaa Miller, naturopath and author,
Aussie Body Diet and Detox Plan, Aussie Body Diet Pty. Ltd.

The pure flavor of fresh young coconut really comes through in this
luxurious drink spiced with cinnamon and maca. Raw honey, if you choose
to use the sweetener to bring out the creamy richness of the coconut,
adds a lovely caramel note.

· ·

Water and flesh of 1 whole
  young Thai coconut (see
  Note), or 1 cup (240 ml)
  coconut water and ½ cup
  (40 g) coconut meat
1 tablespoon maca powder
1 tablespoon chia or hemp
  seeds
½ teaspoon ground cinnamon

Optional:
1 teaspoon raw honey, stevia,
  or other sweetener

Recommended supplements:
1 tablespoon barley grass or
  other greens powder
1 tablespoon Udo's Oil Blend
  or other liquid EFA
  (essential fatty acid)

Blend all the ingredients together. Serve immediately.

Makes one serving.

Note: Look for pale, off-white young Thai coconuts with pointy tops.
To open a young coconut, use a heavy, sharp knife to carefully cut a
square in the top. Pour the coconut water into a container. Use the
knife to split the shell into two halves; scrape the coconut meat out
with a spoon.

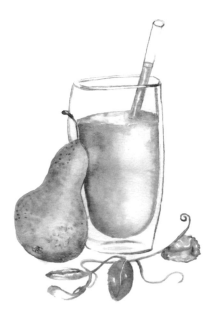

LONDON GREENS
The Juicery

Watercress and basil add a refreshing flavor twist to this green juice,
while coconut water and cucumber provide plenty of hydrating benefits.
Pear is subtly sweet and smoothes out the flavors perfectly.

1 pear
1 cup (50 g) watercress
9 inches (23 cm) cucumber
⅔ cup (160 ml) unsweetened
  coconut water
4 fresh basil leaves

Blend all the ingredients together. Serve immediately.

Makes one serving.

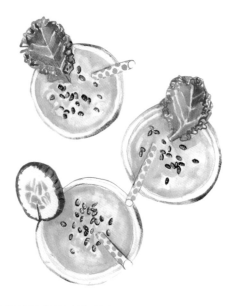

GLOWING GREEN SMOOTHIE
from Amelia Freer, nutritional therapist and founder, Freer Nutrition

Naturally sweet, pure coconut water and fresh apple juice pair
with crisp cucumber, creamy avocado, and textural chia seeds in
this slightly green smoothie. Add a spoonful of spirulina
or pea protein powder for an extra dose of nutrition.

6 inches (15 cm) cucumber
½ avocado
1 apple
Handful organic kale
1 tablespoon chia seeds
1 cup (240 ml) unsweetened
  coconut water

Recommended supplements:
1 tablespoon greens powder
  such as spirulina, or pea
  protein

Blend all the ingredients together. Serve immediately.

Makes one serving.

KEY WEST
AFTER-YOGA SMOOTHIE
from Moises Mehl, nood food Raw Food chef

Nutrient-rich spirulina is paired with creamy avocado and banana and sweet apple to make a deliciously healthful drink. Add a little sweetener and you could call it dessert.

. . . .

1 apple
1 banana
½ avocado

Optional:
Seeds from ½ vanilla bean
  (see Note, page 88)
Raw honey to taste

Blend all the ingredients together. Serve immediately, blended with ice, poured over ice cubes, or at room temperature with no ice.

Makes one serving.

PRE-WORKOUT
GREEN SMOOTHIE
The Juicery

This refreshing shake is perfect as a pre-workout snack. It's a hydrating drink full of phytonutrients and fiber without a lot of heavier protein and fats. It provides all the fuel you need to make it through a workout without weighing you down.

. . . .

½ cup (120 ml) unsweetened
  coconut water
½ banana
½ apple
¾ cup (30 g) spinach
1 romaine leaf
½ cup (25 g) cilantro leaves
¼ lime, peeled
2 ice cubes

Blend all the ingredients together. Serve immediately.

Makes one serving.

DETOX SMOOTHIE
from James Duigan, founder, Bodyism

With cooling cucumber and mint and hydrating coconut water,
this smoothie provides a refreshing hit of nutrition during a detox.

. . . .

1 cup (240 ml) unsweetened
 coconut water
2 large handfuls spinach
1 stalk celery
6 inches (15 cm) cucumber
½ apple
1 teaspoon chopped mint
1 teaspoon grated fresh
 ginger

Recommended supplement:
1 serving greens powder,
 preferably Bodyism

Blend all the ingredients together. Serve immediately,
blended with ice, poured over ice cubes, or at room
temperature with no ice.

Makes one serving.

COCONUT MANGO SMOOTHIE
from Cal-a-Vie

This light and nutty shake, packed with hydrating
electrolytes and muscle-supporting protein, makes a perfect
post-workout pick-me-up.

. . . .

1 cup (240 ml) unsweetened
 coconut water
½ cup (120 ml) nondairy milk
1 cup (180 g) frozen chopped
 mango
½ teaspoon coconut extract

Recommended supplement:
1 serving protein powder

Blend all the ingredients together. Serve immediately.

Makes one serving.

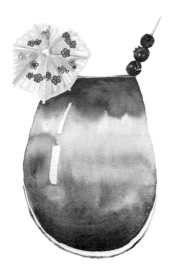

SUNSET SMOOTHIE
The Juicery, The Bloomsbury Hotel

The Sunset Smoothie packs plenty of electrolytes and potassium
to hydrate and replenish, and all the antioxidants protect
your body from free-radical damage and premature aging. The beautiful
drink is also delicious: fresh tasting and just a little sweet.

⅔ cup (160 ml) unsweet-
ened coconut water
½ cup (120 ml) acai and
pomegranate juice, mixed
1 cup (160 g) blueberries
½ banana
3 ice cubes

Blend all the ingredients together. Serve immediately.

Makes one serving.

CARAMBA SMOOTHIE
from Pure Yoga, Hong Kong

This fresh, alkalizing smoothie makes a great pre-yoga drink
(enjoy it about two hours before your exercise routine).
Cilantro has detoxifying, cleansing effects.

1 cup (240 ml) unsweetened
  coconut water
1 cup (170 g) pineapple
2 inches (5 cm) cucumber
1 tablespoon chopped fresh
  cilantro

Blend all the ingredients together. Serve immediately, blended with ice, poured over ice cubes, or at room temperature with no ice.

Makes one serving.

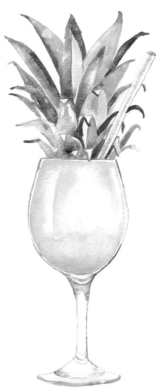

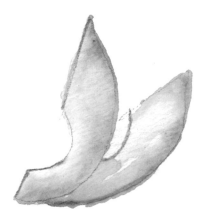

AVOCADO-COCONUT SMOOTHIE

from Abigail James, international facialist and well-being expert

This is a smoothie for your skin: The healthy fats in creamy avocado are great for the skin, parsley is a powerful blood purifier, and coconut water adds a kick of magnesium and the hydration that's vital to skin health.

1 cup (240 ml) unsweetened
  coconut water
1 avocado
2 apples
1 kiwi, peeled
½ lemon, peeled
1 inch (2.5 cm) fresh ginger,
  peeled
5 to 6 sprigs parsley

Recommended supplements:
1 teaspoon MSM powder
1 to 2 teaspoons maca
  powder

Blend all the ingredients together. Serve immediately, blended with ice, poured over ice cubes, or at room temperature with no ice.

Makes one serving.

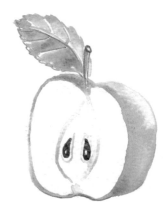

....

THE JAVA

from Lior Lev Sercarz, chef, spice blender, and founder, La Boîte

This unusual smoothie highlights the Borneo N.26 spice blend
with long pepper from Java, Indonesia. It has a great balance between
sweet and acidic notes with a bit of heat and fresh herbaceous flavors.

....

1 Fuji apple, cut into eighths
20 grapes, cut in half
½ cup (120 ml) fresh
  pomegranate juice
1 tablespoon fresh lime juice
1 teaspoon ground Szechuan
  peppercorns or Borneo
  N.26 spice blend
  (available at specialty stores
  or online)
¼ cup (8 g) cilantro leaves
1 cup (240 ml) unsweetened
  coconut water
¼ cup (40 g) pomegranate
  seeds

In a large bowl, combine the apple, grapes,
pomegranate juice, lime juice, and spice blend
and stir well. Cover and refrigerate for 3 hours.

Transfer to a blender, add the cilantro and coconut
water, and blend until smooth. Pour into a chilled
glass, garnish with the pomegranate seeds, and serve
immediately.

Makes one serving.

PROBIOTIC SKIN TONIC
from Julie Elliott, founder, In Fiore

Antioxidants, probiotics, and colostrum help protect the skin from the
inside out. Colostrum provides the body with a wealth of growth factors,
which detoxify and help with cell regeneration. As a result, you'll notice
youthful, nourished, and elastic skin. The tartness of the blueberries
can be offset with a bit of stevia, if you'd like. If you cannot find coconut
water kefir, substitute with unsweetened coconut water.

½ cup (120 ml) coconut
  water kefir
1½ cups ice cubes
¼ cup (40 g) blueberries
2 tablespoons flaxseed oil

Optional:
Raw honey to taste

Recommended supplements:
¼ teaspoon colostrum
¼ teaspoon probiotics
½ teaspoon goji berry powder

Blend all the ingredients together. Serve immediately,

Makes one serving.

STRAWBERRY BANANA ORANGE SMOOTHIE

from Rosa Reisman, author and registered nutritional consultant

A sweet and creamy milkshake-like smoothie loaded with
potassium and antioxidants. A real treat!

. . . .

1 cup (240 ml) milk
½ small banana, sliced
½ cup (80 g) frozen or fresh
  sliced strawberries
1 small orange, peeled
1 tablespoon raw honey
5 ice cubes

Blend all the ingredients together. Serve immediately.

Makes one serving.

EVERYONE LOVES A SUPER BERRY SMOOTHIE

from Schuyler Grant, cocreator, Wanderlust;
director, Kula Yoga Project

Freezing bananas is a great trick for saving those that are quickly
turning brown. Here they help make this berry-rich, antioxidant-packed
smoothie extra creamy and sweet. The yogurt also adds
creaminess and those gut-healthy probiotics as well as protein,
vitamins, and healthy fats.

. . . .

½ banana (preferably frozen
  in chunks)
½ cup (70 g) berries
½ cup (100 g) acai powder
½ cup (120 ml) whole milk
  yogurt
½ cup (120 ml) nut milk,
  preferably homemade
  (pages 84-86)
Ice cubes

Blend all the ingredients together. Serve immediately.

Makes one serving.

Recommended supplement:
½ teaspoon spirulina powder

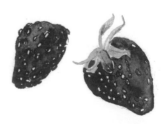

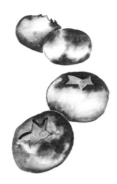

BLUEBERRY BLITZ SMOOTHIE

from Marcelle Pick, R.N.C., M.S.N., OB/GYN N.P.,
best-selling author and cofounder, Women to Women

Nutty almond milk pairs especially well with the bright, fresh tang
of high-protein Greek yogurt and blueberries.

⅔ cup (160 ml) almond nut
milk, preferably homemade
(page 84)
1 cup (150 g) frozen
blueberries
½ cup (90 g) plain Greek
yogurt
4 large kale leaves, tough
stems and ribs removed

Optional:
Raw honey to taste

Blend all the ingredients together. Serve immediately, blended with ice, poured over ice cubes, or at room temperature with no ice.

Makes one serving.

BREAKFAST ENERGIZER
The Juicery

You know it's going to be a good morning when you can start it off with this shake, full of fiber and healthy fats to keep you going. If you use invigorating, slightly sour kefir you'll also get a boost of belly-friendly probiotics.

½ banana
¼ cup (20 g) raw rolled oats
1 tablespoon chia seeds
1 tablespoon almond butter
Pinch ground cinnamon
½ cup (120 ml) kefir or
    almond nut milk, preferably
    homemade (page 84)
Filtered water as needed

Optional:
1 teaspoon raw honey

Blend all the ingredients together, adding water as needed to achieve the desired consistency. Serve immediately, poured over ice cubes, or at room temperature with no ice.

Makes one serving.

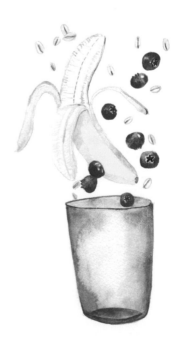

TROPICAL FLORIDA FRUIT SMOOTHIE

from Robert Ciborowski, executive chef, Westin Hotels & Resorts, Walt Disney World Swan and Dolphin Resort

This is one frozen treat that will instantly transport you to a warm, tropical place, because sometimes we need a little sunshine in our glass! And it doesn't hurt that all these tropical fruits are loaded with enzymes, vitamins, and antioxidants. Kids will especially love the oversize ice cube with the floating fruit (specialty stores now sell ice cube molds of many shapes and sizes).

For the ice cube:
¼ cup (25 g) fresh pineapple
¼ cup (25 g) peeled orange segments
¼ cup (25 g) frozen strawberries

1 banana, sliced
⅓ cup (60 g) diced pineapple
⅓ cup (60 g) frozen strawberries
1 mango, peeled, pitted, and diced
¼ cup (90 g) Greek yogurt
5 ice cubes, crushed
Mint leaves

Make the ice cube: Juice the pineapple and pour into a giant ice-cube mold. Freeze for 1 hour. Remove from the freezer. Juice the orange segments. Place the frozen strawberries in the mold and top with the fresh orange juice. Freeze until needed.

Blend the banana, pineapple, strawberries, mango, yogurt, and crushed ice in a high-speed blender until smooth. Serve with the giant ice cube, garnished with mint leaves.

Makes one serving.

SWISS ALP SUMMER MUESLI

from Meghan Telpner, certified nutritional therapist and director,
Academy of Culinary Nutrition

This comforting dish takes eating your whole grains
to a new and delicious level. By soaking your grains, nuts, and seeds
overnight you make them a lot easier to digest, and it's all ready
and waiting for you in the morning.

¼ cup (25 g) dry muesli mix (see Note)
1 tablespoon plain yogurt or fresh lemon juice, or more if needed
Filtered water as needed
½ apple, grated
1 tablespoon ground flaxseed
Ground cinnamon to taste
Raw honey or maple syrup to taste
Fresh fruit

In a small bowl, combine the muesli mix and yogurt, then add enough filtered water to cover the mixture generously. Cover the bowl with a tea towel or plate and let sit on the counter for a minimum of 9 hours or up to 12 hours.

Stir in the apple, flaxseed, cinnamon, honey, fruit, and more water or yogurt to achieve your desired consistency. Serve immediately.

Makes one serving.

Note: To make about 4¼ cups (440 g) muesli mix, combine the following and store in a large jar with a tight lid:

2½ cups (125 g) rolled oats
⅓ cup (80 g) sprouted buckwheat groats or buckwheat flakes
½ cup (75 g) walnut pieces
¼ cup (60 g) hulled pumpkin seeds (pepitas)
¼ cup (60 g) shelled sunflower seeds
¼ cup (40 g) dried cranberries, raisins, and/or chopped dried apricots

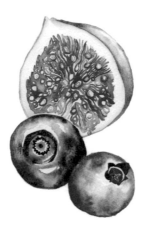

FIG AND HUCKLEBERRY SMOOTHIE
from Julie Elliott, founder, In Fiore

Two unusual ingredients make this milky, tangy smoothie a potent
nutritional surprise. Huckleberries are a great source of vitamins B and C,
which help support and speed up the metabolic rate and keep
skin tone healthy. Cultured buttermilk contains probiotics that promote
healthy digestion—and healthy digestion shows up in clearer,
healthier skin, imparting a natural glow and elasticity.

3 fresh figs
¼ cup (40 g) huckleberries
¼ cup (40 g) blueberries
1 cup (240 ml) buttermilk
1 tablespoon raw honey
1 tablespoon flaxseed oil
4 ice cubes

Optional:
1 egg yolk

Recommended supplement:
1 serving probiotics

Blend all the ingredients together. Serve immediately.

Makes one serving.

Note: Egg yolks act as an emulsifier and add a creamy texture to
smoothies. Nutritionally, yolks contain caratenoids lutein and zeaxanthin, as well as sulfur. All three are essential for production of collagen
and keratin, which results in glowing skin, shiny hair, and strong nails.

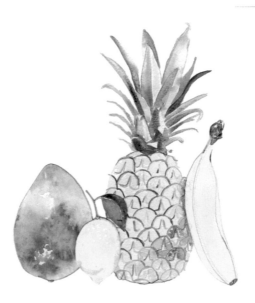

ANANDA SPECIAL
from Ananda in the Himalayas

This creamy, citrusy smoothie loaded with summery tropical
fruit is a true crowd-pleaser. Pineapple contains digestive
enzymes and yogurt provides immune-boosting probiotics,
so here we have a real stomach soother.

½ cup (120 g) pineapple
½ cup (80 g) mango, peeled
  and pitted
½ lemon, peeled
½ (130 g) green apple,
  roughly chopped
½ banana
⅓ cup (20 g) plain yogurt

Optional:
1 tablespoon raw honey

Juice the pineapple, mango, and lemon. Transfer
to a blender, add the apple, banana, yogurt, and honey,
if using, and blend until smooth. Serve immediately,
blended with ice, poured over ice cubes, or at room
temperature with no ice.

Makes one serving.

AVOCADO SMOOTHIE

from Mark Zeitouni, executive chef, Standard Hotel, Miami

Packed with nourishing, rich, healthy fats and the sweet goodness
of apple, this smoothie is the perfect afternoon snack.

½ avocado
¼ cup (60 ml) plain yogurt
1 apple
1 teaspoon vanilla extract
4 to 5 ice cubes
1½ cups (350 ml) filtered
  water
Pinch fine sea salt

Optional:
1 tablespoon maple syrup

Blend all the ingredients together. Serve immediately.

Makes one serving.

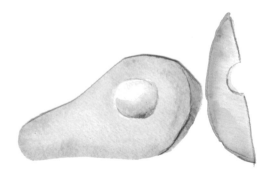

DR. BLUM'S HORMONE-BALANCE BLEND

from Susan Blum, M.D., director, Blum Center for Health
in Rye Brook, NY; author, *The Immune System Recovery Plan*

The ingredients in this drink were handpicked by Dr. Blum for
their ability to help hormonal balance. The cruciferous greens and the
limonene in the white of the lemon peel, as well as the rosemary,
can help your liver do a better job of processing estrogen. Adding protein
powder will make this a meal on its own and help sustain your energy
for hours. Try pumpkin seed powder, rice protein powder, or pure whey
protein powder. Subtly sweet, with an earthy flavor from the
kale and celery, the juice is refreshing and invigorating.

½ apple
1 stalk celery
Handful parsley
Handful cilantro
½ lemon, zest removed (keep
  the white pith on the
  lemon, but peel off the
  yellow part with a vegetable
  peeler)
½ brick frozen acai berry
  puree, or ¼ cup (40 g)
  frozen blueberries
3 large kale leaves
1 sprig rosemary
1 tablespoon flaxseed oil
½ cup (120 ml) cold water,
  or more if needed

Recommended supplement:
1 serving protein powder

Juice the apple, celery, parsley, cilantro, lemon, acai,
kale, and rosemary, then stir in the oil and protein
powder, if using, and add the water until the juice is
your desired consistency. Serve immediately, blended
with ice, poured over ice cubes, or at room temperature
with no ice.

Makes one serving.

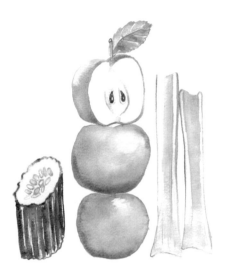

VINE SMOOTHIE

The Juicery

A delicious green drink that combines the best of both worlds:
juiced greens blended with avocado. It's creamy, tart, and jam-packed
with minerals and healthy fats.

2½ green apples
2 stalks celery
8 spinach leaves
½ lime, peeled
1 inch (2.5 cm) cucumber
5 mint leaves
⅓ avocado
5 ice cubes

Juice the apples, celery, spinach, lime, cucumber, and mint. Transfer to a blender and blend in the avocado and ice. Serve immediately.

Makes one serving.

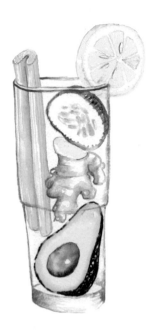

ANTIAGING SMOOTHIE

from James Duigan, founder, Bodyism

Wake up with the spicy heat of ginger, which plays nicely
off the cool cucumber and creamy, rich avocado.
The healthy fats in avocado are anti-inflammatory and
help moisturize and boost your skin from within.

6 inches (15 cm) cucumber
½ avocado
1 stalk celery
Small squeeze fresh lemon
 juice
Small handful greens of
 choice, such as spinach
 or kale
1 teaspoon grated fresh
 ginger
Filtered water as needed

Blend all the ingredients together, adding water as
needed to achieve the desired consistency. Serve
immediately, blended with ice, poured over ice cubes,
or at room temperature with no ice.

Makes one serving.

CHOCO-AVO-NUTTO SMOOTHIE
from Kara Rosen, founder, Plenish Cleanse

This nutty, bittersweet smoothie is a real powerhouse.
It contains high levels of folic acid and other B vitamins
(found in greens), plus loads of antioxidants and nutrients for
stress management (zinc and selenium, found in Brazil
and cashew nuts, can reduce stress).

1 cup (240 ml) cold filtered
  water
½ avocado
½ cup (50 g) packed spinach
  and/or kale
2 teaspoons cashew or Brazil
  nut butter
2 tablespoons cacao nibs
1 teaspoon flaxseed oil or
  chia seed oil
4 ice cubes

Optional:
Molasses to taste

Blend all the ingredients together. Serve immediately, blended with ice, poured over ice cubes, or at room temperature with no ice.

Makes one serving.

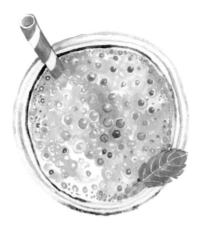

GRATIFYING GREEN SMOOTHIE

from Shonali Sabherwal, macrobiotic nutritionist, chef,
instructor, and founder, Soulfood India

Get your daily dose of greens from this refreshing, sweet smoothie.
The surprising addition of smoky ground cumin is a nod to savory
Indian hot-weather drinks.

1 apple
1 cup (240 ml) filtered water
1 cup (100 g) bean sprouts
2 teaspoons fresh lemon juice
½ teaspoon ground cumin

Optional:
1 banana

Recommended supplements:
1 teaspoon wheatgrass powder
1 teaspoon spirulina powder

Blend the apple, water, and banana, if using, then stir
in the bean sprouts, lemon juice, cumin, and wheatgrass powder and spirulina, if using. Serve immediately,
blended with ice, poured over ice cubes, or at room
temperature with no ice.

Makes one serving.

MANGO CLEANSER SMOOTHIE

from Meghan Telpner, certified nutritionist and director,
Academy of Culinary Nutrition

A creamy smoothie packed with the tropical flavors of mango
and coconut. Great for cleansing the cells of heavy metals, it is also
rich in vitamin C for immunity and skin health.

1 cup (164 g) fresh or frozen
mango
½ cup (20 g) chopped
parsley
6 inches (15 cm) cucumber
1 tablespoon shredded,
unsweetened coconut,
or ½ cup (40 g) grated
fresh young coconut meat
1 teaspoon chopped fresh
ginger
8 ice cubes
1 cup (240 ml) filtered water
or chilled peppermint tea

Recommended supplement:
1 serving protein powder, or
3 tablespoons hemp seeds

Blend all the ingredients together. Serve immediately.

Makes one serving.

LIME AND MINT AGUA FRESCA
from Vitamix

An absolutely refreshing and festive drink. The cucumber and
the mint are cooling, and the melon is hydrating and replenishing.
A perfect drink for a summer fiesta or a lazy siesta . . .

¼ cup (60 ml) filtered water
1 tablespoon raw honey
¾ cup (130 g) diced honeydew melon
¾ cup (100 g) cucumber
¼ lime, peeled
1 tablespoon mint leaves
¼ teaspoon grated lime zest
4 ice cubes

Blend all the ingredients together in a high-speed
blender, starting on low speed and gradually
increasing to high speed until very smooth; use a
tamper or large blender-safe spoon, if needed.
Serve immediately.

Makes one serving.

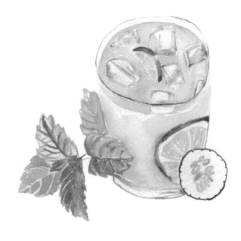

SPICY PIÑA COLADA
from David Laris, founder, David Laris Creates

Tart-sweet, fresh-pressed juice loaded with healthful fruits and vegetables
and a hit of fresh ginger is blended with smooth avocado and cool mint
(and ice, if you want a frosty drink) in this refreshing, easy-to-love shake.

. . . .

2 large stalks celery
1 large carrot
2 rings pineapple
1 green apple
½ lime, peeled
1½ tablespoons chopped
  fresh ginger
½ avocado
1 teaspoon minced mint

Juice the celery, carrot, pineapple, apple, lime, and
ginger. Transfer to a blender and add the avocado and
mint. Blend until smooth. Serve immediately, blended
with ice, poured over ice cubes, or at room temperature
with no ice.

Makes one serving.

GREEN ANTI-INFLAMMATORY
PIÑA COLADA
from Meghan Telpner, certified nutritionist and director,
Academy of Culinary Nutrition

With green tea for energy and antioxidants and pineapple for sweetness
and a boost of enzymes, this shake has anti-inflammatory benefits
and is great post-workout or when you're healing from an injury.

. . . .

Handful spinach
½ frozen zucchini
1 tablespoon shredded,
  unsweetened coconut,
  or ½ cup (40 g) grated,
  fresh young coconut meat
1 cup (165 g) fresh or frozen
  pineapple
Juice of ½ lime
8 ice cubes
1 cup (240 ml) chilled green
  tea

Recommended supplement:
1 serving protein powder, or
  3 tablespoons hemp seeds

Blend all the ingredients together. Serve immediately.

Makes one serving.

ICED BLUEBERRY SHOT

from Hala El-Shafie, founder, Nutrition Rocks

These amazing little shots are so simple to make and to multiply depending on how many shots you want. Try one first thing in the morning to get your day started or as a cool pick-me-up in midafternoon.

5 blueberries
2 ice cubes

Blend the ingredients together. Serve immediately.

Makes one serving.

LEAFY GREENS SMOOTHIE

from Vitamix

Swiss chard is loaded with phytonutrients and chlorophyll. Combined with vitamin C from the orange and the refreshing sweetness from the grapes, this nutrient powerhouse will go down easy.

¼ cup (40 g) green grapes
¼ orange, peeled
¼ apple
1 cup (40 g) Swiss chard
8 ice cubes

Blend all the ingredients together in a high-speed blender, starting on low speed and gradually increasing to high speed until very smooth; use a tamper, or large blender-safe spoon, if needed. Serve immediately.

Makes one serving.

NEW YORK MINUTE

from Dr. David Colbert, founder and head physician,
New York Dermatology Group; founder, Colbert MD Skincare

Looking for a real energy boost on a hectic day? Try this caffeinated drink,
with energizing and stamina-building goji berries, and vitamin E, which
boosts your immune response and the negative effects of stress.

¼ cup (60 g) goji berries
1 tablespoon raw honey
½ cup (120 ml) brewed
  Arabica coffee, cooled
1 cup (240 ml) filtered
  water
1 serving vitamin E oil
  (or 1 vitamin E capsule,
  opened)

Blend all the ingredients together. Serve at room
temperature or over ice.

Makes one serving.

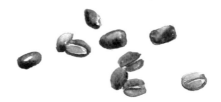

SHIBUI CUCUMBER CORDIAL
from Cristina Paradelo, Shibui Spa at the Greenwich Hotel

Who said cocktails must contain liquor? This combination
is wildly refreshing, with a little kick of ginger to keep
things interesting. It doesn't hurt that it's also anti-inflammatory
and does wonders for your skin!

12 inches (30 cm) cucumber
¼ inch fresh ginger
3 or 4 ice cubes
2 tablespoons pure yuzu juice
(available through specialty
stores)
Cold sparkling water

Optional:
1 tablespoon raw honey

Juice the cucumber and ginger. Add the ice cubes,
then stir in the yuzu juice and honey, if using; top off
with sparkling water. Serve immediately.

Makes one serving.

GINGER GREEN TEA ELIXIR
from Nini Ordoubadi, founder, Tay Tea

Ginger is a potent anti-inflammatory herb that also helps
get the digestive juices flowing and quells nausea and stomach
upset. Here it's combined with green tea—an antioxidant
powerhouse—and naturally sweetened with fruit.

4 to 6 thin slices peeled fresh
  ginger
1 cup (240 ml) filtered water
Juice of ½ lime, or more to
  taste
1 to 2 tablespoons white grape
  juice, or more to taste
2 tablespoons sencha green
  tea leaves or genmaicha tea
½ cup (80 g) cantaloupe

Put the ginger and ½ cup (120 ml) water in a small
saucepan and bring to a boil. Lower the heat and
simmer for 10 to 20 minutes (use more ginger and boil
longer for a spicier tea). Remove from the heat and
add the lime juice and grape juice to taste.

Put the tea leaves in a heatproof container and pour
½ cup (120 ml) boiling water over them. Steep for
10 minutes, then strain into the ginger tea. Let cool,
then chill in the refrigerator for 1 hour. Transfer to a
blender, add the cantaloupe, and blend until smooth.
Serve immediately, blended with ice, poured over ice
cubes, or at room temperature with no ice.

Makes one serving.

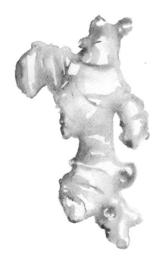

PEACH PARTY

from Katrine van Wyk, author and holistic health coach;
nutrition consultant, The Juicery

Sweet ripe peaches are sure winners with kids.
The almond milk and the flaxseeds add creaminess to this
dairy-free drink—and some healthy fats, too.

· ·

1 cup (240 ml) almond nut
   milk, preferably homemade
   (page 84)
1 cup (150 g) fresh or frozen
   peaches
1 tablespoon flaxseeds
3 ice cubes

Blend all the ingredients together. Serve immediately.

Makes one serving.

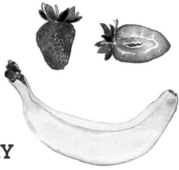

STRAWBERRY CREAM

from Katrine van Wyk, author and holistic health coach;
nutrition consultant, The Juicery

With a taste and color similar to strawberry ice cream, the kids
will be asking for this smoothie all the time! Coconut milk is rich in the
healthy fats that are so important for active, growing kids and is
a great alternative to dairy. But go ahead: Call it a milkshake.

· ·

1 cup (240 ml) unsweetened
   coconut milk, preferably
   homemade (page 88)
1 cup (170 g) fresh or frozen
   strawberries
1 banana
½ cup (120 ml) filtered water

Blend all the ingredients together. Serve immediately.

Makes one serving.

BERRY BLIZZARD

from Katrine van Wyk, author and holistic health coach;
nutrition consultant, The Juicery

A mixed berry smoothie never fails, sweet and delicious and packed
with protective antioxidants. Sneak in a cup of spinach, too,
but don't worry: The kids won't even know it's there. The dark color
from the berries and the sweetness of the banana hide it well.

. . . .

1 cup (150 g) frozen mixed
   berries
1½ cups (350 ml) unsweet-
   ened coconut water
1 cup (40 g) spinach
½ banana
1 teaspoon chia seeds

Blend all the ingredients together. Serve immediately.

Makes one serving.

MANGO LASSI

from Katrine van Wyk, author and holistic health coach;
nutrition consultant, The Juicery

Lassis are cooling Indian drinks that are perfect on hot summer days.
The yogurt adds some protein and healthy probiotics, and
the dash of cardamom makes this sweet and easy-to-love drink
a little adventurous and exotic.

. . . .

½ cup (120 ml) plain full-fat
   yogurt
½ cup (120 ml) filtered
   water
1½ cups (250 g) mangos
1 tablespoon raw honey
Pinch ground cardamom
3 ice cubes

Blend all the ingredients together. Serve immediately.

Makes one serving.

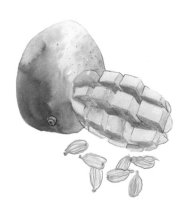

GREEN PEA SOUP

from Martynka Wawrzyniak, Rizzoli book editor

Green peas are the perfect spring food: deliciously sweet, grassy,
and oh-so-creamy when blended into a soup. This version is super-quick
and easy to make, yet wonderfully satisfying. The coconut oil adds a nice
nutty sweetness to the dish, but also healthy medium-chain fatty acids that
can actually help you lose weight! For a chilled summer version of this soup,
omit the cayenne and add a large handful of mint leaves, blend,
then chill until cold before serving.

10 ounces (280 g) organic
  frozen green peas
1 cup (240 ml) boiling water
1 tablespoon coconut oil or
  coconut butter
Pinch fine sea salt
Fresh lemon juice to taste

Optional:
Pinch ground cayenne
Handful baby spinach leaves,
  or 1 teaspoon greens
  powder or spirulina powder

Put the peas in a colander and pour the boiling water
over them to thaw them quickly, then transfer the peas
to a high-speed blender, along with the remaining
ingredients. Blend, starting at low speed and gradually
increasing to high speed, until slightly warmed, frothy,
and silky smooth. Blend longer if you want it hotter.

Makes one serving.

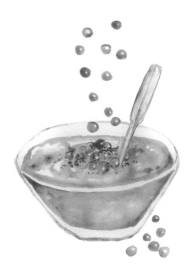

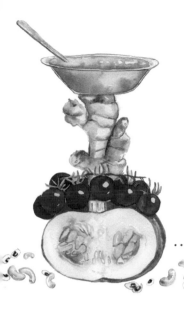

KABOCHA HERBAL BROTH
from Jess Ng, founder, ReOrient

By slowly simmering these nutritious foods you can draw some of the healthful minerals and vitamins out into the liquid broth. It's a perfect soothing and healing addition to any cleanse or when you're a little under the weather, as it's packed with antioxidants and anti-inflammatory benefits. Look for dried tangerine peel in Chinese herbal shops and grocery stores, where it's called *chen pi*. If you want to eat the black-eyed peas, soak them overnight in water to cover before using them in this recipe; otherwise, just enjoy the broth and strain out the beans themselves.

¼ cup (30 g) raw cashews
¼ cup (60 g) dried black-eyed peas
1 slice dried tangerine peel (see headnote)
3 slices fresh ginger
10 cups (2.4 liter) filtered water
2 teaspoons dried goji berries
1½ pounds (680 g) kabocha squash (about ½ squash), seeded and cut into 1-inch (2.5-cm) pieces
2 large tomatoes, quartered
A few drops extra-virgin olive oil

Optional:
Fine sea salt to taste

Rinse the cashews, black-eyed peas, and tangerine peel and drain. Put in a pot and add the ginger and water. Bring to a boil over high heat, then lower the heat and simmer for 25 minutes.

Rinse the goji berries and add them to the pot, along with the squash, tomatoes, and oil. Bring to a boil, then simmer for 30 minutes, or until the squash and tomatoes are very tender and have melted into the broth. Pour through a fine-mesh sieve into a bowl and serve the broth warm, seasoned with salt if you like.

Makes four servings.

WHITE GAZPACHO

from Bobbi Neal, hospitality consultant and founder, The Joint Cafe

Cauliflower belongs to the *brassica* family of vegetables, which are known for their preventative health benefits. Pine nuts are packed with healthy fats and make this soup deliciously creamy, with a nutty flavor.

½ head cauliflower
2 slices multigrain bread, crusts removed
¼ cup (30 g) pine nuts, toasted
2 cloves garlic, chopped
2 tablespoons sherry vinegar
1 large shallot, chopped
6 inches (15 cm) cucumber, peeled and chopped
Pinch fine sea salt

For garnish:
¼ cup (40 g) finely diced cucumber
¼ cup (30 g) slivered almonds
Drizzle extra-virgin olive oil

In a food processor or blender, combine the cauliflower, bread, pine nuts, garlic, vinegar, shallot, and chopped cucumber and puree until very smooth. Taste and season with salt. Transfer to a bowl, cover, and refrigerate until completely chilled, at least 30 minutes. Ladle into chilled serving bowls, garnish with the finely diced cucumber and slivered almonds, drizzle with the oil, and serve. For a gluten-free version, replace bread with a double portion of pine nuts.

Makes two servings.

THE ALKALIZER

from Shonali Sabherwal, macrobiotic nutritionist, chef,
instructor, and founder, Soulfood India

Cucumber is alkalizing, and so strengthens the blood.
Coconut milk brings good saturated fat to the table, and also burns
into energy, providing a natural boost. Cilantro is known to regulate
blood-sugar levels and aid digestion, making this a great savory soup
to enjoy toward the end of a day of heavier meals.

12 inches (30 cm) cucumber
1 clove garlic, chopped, or
   more to taste
1 cup (240 ml) vegetable stock
1 cup (240 ml) unsweetened
   coconut milk, preferably
   homemade (page 88)
1 tablespoon fresh lime juice
1 tablespoon minced cilantro
Fine sea salt

Blend the cucumber, garlic, and stock until smooth,
then add the coconut milk, lime juice, cilantro, and salt
to taste and blend until smooth. Refrigerate until completely chilled, at least 30 minutes. Serve cold.

Makes two servings.

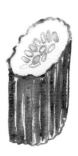

GO-TO GREEN SOUP (OR SMOOTHIE)

from Jasmine and Melissa Hemsley, founders, HEMSLEY + HEMSLEY; authors, *The Art of Eating Well*

This is a great smoothie or soup to whip up when you're craving something green and light. Include the savory ingredients—garlic, cayenne, and so on—for a spicier soup that feels like more of a main course. Dulse seaweed is rich in iodine and adds a touch of umami salinity to the soup.

Pinch dried dulse
1¼ cups (300 ml) filtered water, or more as needed
1 to 2 green apples
6 inches (15 cm) cucumber
2 celery sticks
2 lightly packed cups (70 g) spinach or kale, kale stems removed
½ large avocado
½ cup (20 g) watercress
1 inch (2.5 cm) fresh ginger, peeled and chopped
¼ cup (10 g) fresh parsley
3 tablespoons fresh lemon juice
1 teaspoon supergreens powder such as chlorella or spirulina

Optional savory ingredients:
2 scallions
1 medium to large clove garlic
Tiny pinch cayenne pepper
Pinch fine sea salt

For garnish:
Diced cucumber or chopped fresh parsley
Freshly ground black pepper
Olive oil

Put the dulse in a blender with the water to soak while you prep the rest of the vegetables.

Roughly chop the apples, cucumber, celery, spinach, avocado, watercress, and parsley and add them to the blender, along with all the remaining ingredients except the garnishes. Pulse a few times, then blend until smooth. Add more water as necessary to achieve your desired consistency and serve in glasses at room temperature, or as a soup in bowls at room temperature or warmed gently on the stove in colder weather. Garnish the soup, if you'd like, with some diced cucumber or chopped fresh parsley, black pepper, and a drizzle of oil.

Makes three servings.

CANTALOUPE SOUP

from Dr. Frank Lipman, founder and director,
Eleven Eleven Wellness Center & Be Well

Sweet, spicy, tart, with the flowery scent of basil: It doesn't get much
simpler or more delicious than this cold soup. Use a good-quality fruity
olive oil so its flavor comes through.

1 cantaloupe, peeled, seeded,
   and chopped
Juice of 1 lime
1 tablespoon extra-virgin
   olive oil
½ teaspoon crushed red
   pepper flakes
Pinch fine sea salt
Fresh basil leaves

In a food processor, combine the cantaloupe, lime
juice, oil, red pepper flakes, and salt. Pulse until not
quite pureed—there should still be small chunks of
cantaloupe in the mixture.

Pour half of the mixture into a bowl, then puree the
rest until very smooth. Pour the smooth puree into the
chunky puree and stir. Cover and refrigerate until completely chilled, at least 30 minutes. Ladle into chilled
serving bowls. Garnish with basil and serve.

Makes four to six servings.

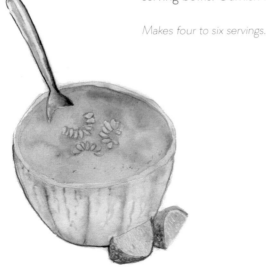

FRESH
+
CREAMY

Acai + Banana + Berries
Avocado + Greens + Banana
Blueberry + Vanilla
Cherry + Almond + Vanilla
Mango + Peach
Mango + Tangerine
Pineapple + Papaya
Spinach + Banana
Strawberry + Banana + Vanilla
Strawberry + Orange

RICH
+
TANGY

Acai + Cacao
Apple + Cinnamon
Avocado + Spinach + Peach
Cacao + Banana
Kiwi + Avocado
Mango + Yogurt
Mixed Berries + Yogurt

NUTTY
+
SWEET

Almond + Apricot
Almond + Date + Maca
Banana + Almond + Cacao
Banana + Peanut Butter
Banana + Walnut
Banana + Coconut
Blueberry + Almond
Cacao + Nut Milk
Cacao + Vanilla + Almond
Carrot + Almond + Cardamom
Cashew Milk + Cinnamon + Vanilla + Date
Fig + Almond
Green Tea + Almond Milk + Dates
Mixed Berries + Nut Milk
Peach + Vanilla + Almond
Raspberry + Cacao + Almond
Strawberry + Almond + Coconut

TART
+
CREAMY

Banana + Spinach
Cacao + Cherry
Cherry + Mixed Berry
Orange + Plum
Raspberry + Goji

REFRESHING
+
LUSCIOUS

Blueberry + Banana
Cacao + Avocado
Coconut + Spinach + Banana
Kale + Apple + Almond
Lime + Coconut + Banana
Mango + Coconut
Orange + Kale
Papaya + Yogurt
Peach + Coconut Milk
Pear + Avocado
Pineapple + Coconut Milk
Strawberry + Yogurt

FRESH
+
CLEAN

Acai + Spinach
Avocado + Cucumber
Beet + Mixed Berries
Greens + Banana + Coconut
Hibiscus + Raspberries
Kiwi + Pear + Greens
Peach + Kale
Pineapple + Cilantro
Tomato + Spinach + Olive Oil

FLAVOR COMBINATIONS
SMOOTHIES

There are thousands of combinations
of fruits, vegetables, herbs, nut milks, and other
liquids that together make delicious smoothies.
Here are some of our favorites that can be used
as bases for your own recipes. Experiment!

GREEN
+
SPICY

Greens + Honeydew Melon + Jalapeño
Greens + Coconut
Kale + Cacao
Kale + Pineapple
Mango + Greens + Cilantro
Papaya + Spinach + Lime

COOLING
+
CRISP

Blueberry + Oats + Yogurt
Cacao + Mint
Green Tea + Lime
Mixed Berries + Greens
Tomato + Basil + Watermelon

SPICY
+
SWEET

Carrot + Ginger + Apple
Mango + Ginger
Orange + Ginger

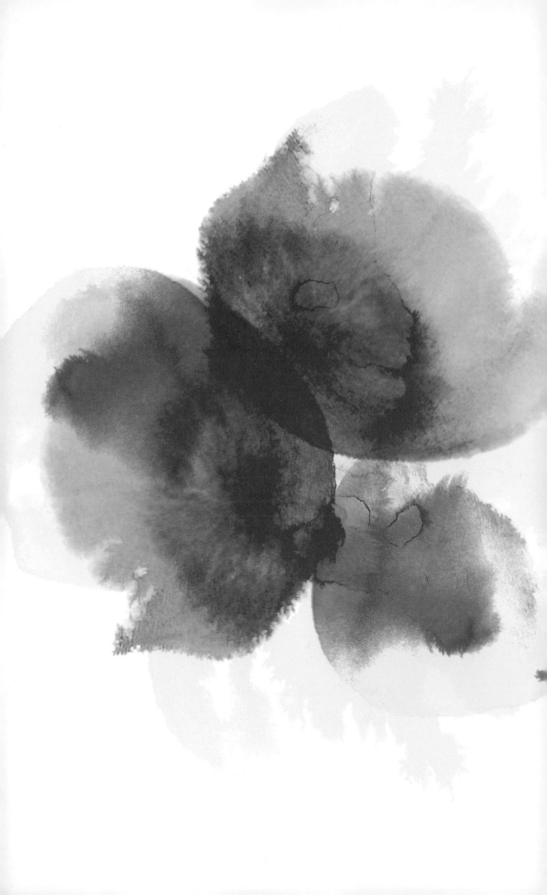

ICED TEAS, WARM INFUSIONS, & SPARKLING DRINKS

It's easy to fall into a rut when it comes to everyday drinks—we have our favorite hot teas, simple (but easily addictive) sodas, maybe a basic iced tea or lemonade when the weather warms. The recipes here will greatly expand your repertoire and open up a whole world of possibilities for seasonal drinks with a healthy twist.

Hot drinks—some with caffeine, some very low in caffeine, and some free of it altogether— are made with fresh seasonal ingredients, interesting combinations of spices, and fragrant herbs. They will warm your body, provide immune support during cold and flu season, and soothe your soul throughout the long winter months.

The special iced teas and sparkling sodas, bubbly with sparkling water or, if you can find it, sparkling coconut water, will be welcome additions to your drinks rotation. They wouldn't be out of place at a cocktail party mixed with a small-batch vodka or gin or a great champagne (and on their own they'd be a creative nonalcoholic option) or enjoyed garden or poolside. These are fun, refreshing, invigorating drinks to get you through a warm, lazy afternoon or to share with friends after hours.

RED ICED TEA YEOTINI

from Michelle Ngoh, cofounder, Yeotown

A refreshing, slightly sweet and tart drink with great
calming benefits for the belly.

1⅓ cups (320 ml) filtered
water
2 rosehip tea bags
1 sprig mint, plus more as
desired
⅔ cup (150 g) crushed or
juiced raspberries
Juice of ½ lime

Optional:
Coconut sugar

Bring the water to a boil and pour it over the tea bags
and the sprig of mint in a teapot. Let steep for a few
minutes, then add more mint, the raspberries, and
lime juice; stir in coconut sugar to taste, if you like. Let
cool, then discard the tea bags and serve in a glass over
plenty of ice.

Makes one serving.

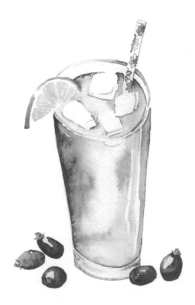

CUCUMBER MOJITO TEA DIGESTIF

from Jasmine and Melissa Hemsley, founders, HEMSLEY + HEMSLEY;
authors, *The Art of Eating Well*

Perfect to serve in small doses as a digestif after a meal or between courses
to cleanse the palate, this zingy and refreshing tea has a natural fizz from the
kombucha and an energy boost from the matcha. And you won't miss
the refined sugar or alcohol in this refreshing tippler.

6 inches (15 cm) cucumber,
  cubed
1 tablespoon fresh lime juice
16 large mint leaves
½ teaspoon matcha
  (green tea) powder
1 cup (240 ml) brewed
  kombucha, chilled, or
  more to taste
¼ cup (60 ml) filtered water

Blend the cucumber, lime juice, mint, and matcha until
smooth. Stir in the kombucha and water and serve in a
small glass over ice.

Makes one serving.

· ·

ICED HIBISCUS TEA

from Hala El-Shafie, founder, Nutrition Rocks

Hibiscus tea is made from the fleshy, dark burgundy calyces of the
hibiscus flower, which when dried look like blossoms themselves.
Look for it in Latin American grocery stores, where it might be labeled
"jamaica." The tea is tart and bracing, here subtly sweetened with blueberries;
you can add a few drops of liquid stevia if you'd like.

· ·

Heaping ½ cup (110 g) dried hibiscus
7 cups (1.7 liter) filtered water
1 cup (150 g) fresh or frozen blueberries
1 to 2 tablespoons fresh lime juice

Optional:
Liquid stevia

Put the dried hibiscus in a large heat- and stain-proof container. Bring 4 cups (880 ml) of the water to a boil and pour it over the hibiscus. Let steep for 25 minutes.

Meanwhile, put the blueberries, lime juice, and the remaining 3 cups (710 ml) water in a blender. Blend until very smooth. Slowly pour through a fine-mesh sieve into a serving pitcher; discard the solids and rinse the sieve.

Pour the hibiscus tea through the sieve into the serving pitcher. Stir well and add stevia to taste if needed. Cover and refrigerate until completely chilled, at least 30 minutes. Serve over ice.

Makes two servings.

GINGER LEMON TONIC

from Christina Agnew and Clare Neill, cofounders, Radiance

This spicy lemon tonic—lightly sweetened with maple syrup—
makes an energizing and cleansing start to your day. In the summer,
add ice cubes and enjoy it as a refreshing and alkalizing way
to quench your thirst. In the winter, use only half the cold water and top
it off with boiling water for a warming tonic. Turmeric has powerful
anti-inflammatory properties and is great for your skin and immune system.
The black pepper actually greatly increases your body's absorption
of the active agent in turmeric, called curcumin.

Juice of 2 lemons
1⅔ cups (390 ml) cold filtered
  water, or half cold and half
  boiling
4 teaspoons maple syrup
3 tablespoons minced fresh
  ginger
¼ teaspoon ground cinnamon
Pinch ground turmeric
Tiny pinch freshly ground
  black pepper

Combine all the ingredients and mix or shake well.
Serve immediately, warm or cold, blended with ice,
poured over ice cubes, or at room temperature with
no ice.

Makes one serving.

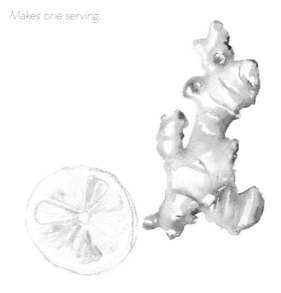

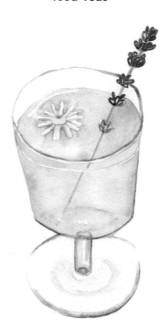

PETAL TEA

from Ananda in the Himalayas

This mild floral tea is calming and cool—perfect for a relaxing summer afternoon on the porch.

¼ cup (30 g) dried chopped lemongrass

5 teaspoons (5 g) dried lavender

1 teaspoon (5 g) dried rose hips

1 teaspoon (3 g) dried red clover

1 teaspoon (3 g) dried chamomile blossoms

4 cups (880 ml) boiling filtered water

Combine all the herbs in a heatproof container and pour the boiling water over them. Let steep for 1 hour, then strain through a fine-mesh sieve and refrigerate until completely chilled, at least 30 minutes. Serve cold.

Makes four servings.

APPLE LEMON BEET ICED TEA

from Alex Probyn, founder, Blends for Friends

Tea and juice are such great sources of antioxidants, and this drink combines them both. The fruits and vegetables are also loaded with some great detox-boosting nutrients and lots of energizing vitamins.

. . . .

1 teaspoon green tea leaves, or 1 green tea bag
½ cup (120 ml) boiling filtered water, plus 1 cup (240 ml) cold
3 small or 2 large apples, peeled
Juice of ½ lemon
1 small beet

Put the tea leaves in a mug and pour the boiling water over them; steep for 3 minutes, then strain into a blender. Add the apples, lemon juice, and beet and blend until smooth. Add the 1 cup cold water and blend again. Serve over ice.

Makes two servings.

ROOIBOS MIXER

from Alex Probyn, founder, Blends for Friends

An antioxidant-loaded, soothing drink with bold, delicious flavor, perfect for an afternoon cuppa. Licorice root is an herb known for its calming effect on the digestive system and has been found to help stimulate defense mechanisms that prevent stomach ulcers. Chile and ginger add some heat and spice that help boost the metabolism and fight inflammation.

. . . .

2 heaping teaspoons rooibos tea leaves, or 2 rooibos tea bags
1 cup (240 ml) boiling filtered water
1 inch (2.5 cm) licorice root, finely ground (½ teaspoon)
6 chili seeds, finely ground
1 tablespoon raw cacao nibs, finely ground, or 1 tablespoon carob powder
3 inches (7 cm) fresh ginger
2 cups (470 ml) cold filtered water, or 2 to 3 cups (470 to 710 ml) hot almond (page 84), rice, or dairy milk
4 ice cubes

Steep the tea in boiling water for 5 minutes, then strain into a pitcher. Stir in the ground licorice root, chili seeds, and cacao nibs. Juice the ginger and add it to the tea. Whisk well, then whisk in the cold water or hot milk. Serve cold over ice or hot.

Makes two servings.

CHERRY AND BERRY ICED TEA

from Alex Probyn, founder, Blends for Friends

Load up on disease-fighting antioxidants with this exceptional concoction of raspberries, strawberries, and sea buckthorn berries. Refreshing, tart, and energizing!

1 teaspoon black tea leaves, or 1 black tea bag (regular or Earl Grey)
½ cup (120 ml) boiling filtered water, plus 1 cup (240 ml) cold
1 heaping tablespoon blueberries
1 heaping tablespoon pitted cherries
1 heaping tablespoon strawberries
1 heaping tablespoon sea buckthorn berries, fresh or frozen, or juice of ½ lemon

Put the tea leaves in a mug and pour the boiling water over them; steep for 3 minutes, then strain into a blender. Add the blueberries, cherries, strawberries, and sea buckthorn berries and blend until smooth. Add the 1 cup cold water and blend again. Serve over ice.

Makes two servings.

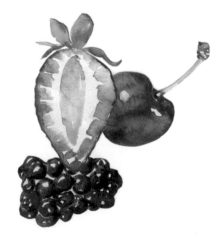

ANTIOXIDANT COFFEE CREAM

from Cristiana Arcangeli, founder, Beauty'In

Can you imagine a better way to boost your morning coffee
than with heart-healthy almond milk, antioxidant-rich berries
and cacao, and blood-sugar–stabilizing cinnamon?
Nope—didn't think so!

½ cup (70 g) mixed berries
2 tablespoons acai juice
½ tablespoon Brazil nuts
Raw honey to taste
½ cup (120 ml) hot brewed
coffee
½ cup (120 ml) almond nut
milk, preferably homemade
(page 84), foam from boiling
milk, reserved
1 tablespoon cacao nibs
Ground cinnamon

In a small bowl, combine the berries, acai juice, nuts,
and honey; transfer to a beautiful drinking glass. In a
blender, blend the coffee, almond milk, and cacao
nibs until smooth, then pour the mixture into the glass.
Spoon the reserved milk foam over the top, sprinkle
with cinnamon, and serve.

Makes one serving.

LOTUS ROOT TEA
from SHA Wellness Clinic

Lotus root is well known for its capacity to help clear respiratory passages,
and is great for people with asthma or those with a cold or the flu.
(Try putting a bit of dried lotus root in brothy soups in cold and flu season.)
This warm infusion is savory and comforting, whether you're in need
of restoration or not.

1 teaspoon ground, dried lotus
root, or 3 or 4 pieces whole
dried lotus root
1 or 2 cups (240 to 470 ml)
filtered water
Pinch fine sea salt
Shoyu to taste

If using ground lotus, put it in a small saucepan with
1 cup (240 ml) water, the salt, and shoyu and heat over
medium heat until the liquid is steaming; do not let it
boil. Serve hot.

If using whole pieces of dried lotus root, put them in
a small saucepan with 2 cups (470 ml) water, bring to
a boil, and boil for about 15 minutes. Discard the roots,
add the salt and shoyu, and serve hot.

Makes one serving.

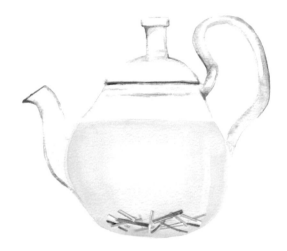

HERB TEA

from Michelle Roques-O'Neil, aromatherapist, healer,
spiritual life coach, and natural perfumer

This is a delicious, energizing, and cleansing tea. Rose is detoxifying
for the liver; lemon verbena is calming and great for digestion;
damiana is a wonderful antidote to lack of energy or libido; and licorice
improves the flow of the spleen, helping release excess fluid and toxins.
Cool spearmint aids digestion. Damiana is a plant that's been used
in Mexico for centuries as a libido booster and aphrodisiac. It helps
increase energy and overall well-being.

2 teaspoons dried lemon
   verbena
1½ teaspoons dried pink
   rosebuds
1 teaspoon dried spearmint
Pinch dried licorice root
Pinch damiana
½ cup (120 ml) boiling filtered
   water

Combine all the ingredients, except the boiling water,
in a bowl and transfer to a jar with lid. Store in a sealed
jar in a cool, dark spot. To brew, put about 1 tablespoon
in a tea bag or infuser in a mug and pour the boiling
water over the tea. Let steep for a few minutes, then
serve hot.

Makes 10 cups of tea.

GREEN COCO TEA

from Brenners Park Hotel and Spa

Hot matcha tea is a luscious and delicious way to enjoy all the
antioxidant benefits of green tea. In this version, you'll use coconut milk,
which is packed with healthy fats that actually boost weight loss!

1 cup (240 ml) hot brewed
matcha green tea
½ cup (120 ml) unsweetened
coconut milk, preferably
homemade (page 88), heated
Raw honey to taste

Stir all the ingredients together in a large mug and
serve hot.

Makes one serving.

WARM SPICY APPLE CARROT JUICE

from David Frenkiel and Luise Vindahl, authors,
Green Kitchen Stories blog

This warm spiced juice may take you straight back to beloved childhood apple-picking outings and the sweet mulled cider that would be your reward on a crisp fall day. It's not as sweet, though, and the carrot and fresh ginger give it an interesting underlayer of flavor, making it a decidedly grown-up cool-weather drink.

About 6 apples
2 carrots
1 inch (2.5 cm) fresh ginger, or more to taste
1 cinnamon stick
2 star anise
2 allspice berries
½ teaspoon cardamom seeds
½ teaspoon ground cinnamon
½ teaspoon freshly grated nutmeg

Juice enough apples to yield 2 cups (470 ml) juice. Juice the carrots and ginger separately.

Put the apple juice, cinnamon stick, star anise, allspice, and cardamom in a saucepan and bring to a boil over high heat. Lower the heat and simmer for 1 to 2 minutes. Remove from the heat, cover, and let steep for 5 to 10 minutes. Pour through a fine-mesh sieve into a heat-proof measuring cup. Stir in the carrot and ginger juice, then pour into serving glasses, sprinkle with ground cinnamon and nutmeg, and serve warm.

Makes two servings.

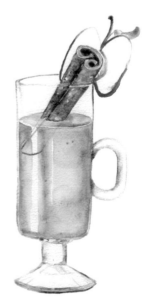

HAWTHORN HIBISCUS ELIXIR

from Jess Ng, founder, ReOrient

A fragrant, delicious, and deeply red drink that soothes both body and mind. Hibiscus has a light blood-pressure-lowering effect, licorice soothes the tummy, and hawthorn is said to relax the heart.

6 cups (1.4 liter) filtered water
Peel of 1 Meyer lemon
Raw honey
1½ teaspoons dried hawthorn berries
1 teaspoon dried hibiscus
½ teaspoon dried licorice root
1 star anise

In a small saucepan, bring 1 cup (240 ml) of the water and the lemon peel to a simmer, cover, and cook until the peel is translucent and the water is flavorful and bitter, 15 to 30 minutes. Add honey to taste. Pour through a fine-mesh sieve into a heat-proof measuring cup and set aside. (Save the peels, which can be dried: candied lemon peel!)

Rinse the hawthorn berries, hibiscus, licorice root, and star anise. Put in a saucepan, add the remaining 5 cups (1.2 liter) water, and bring to a boil over hight heat. Lower the heat to medium and cook for 5 minutes, then remove from the heat and steep for 10 minutes. Strain and add ½ cup (120 ml) of the lemon syrup, or to taste. Serve warm.

Makes four servings.

PURE ALTITUDE INFUSION
from Les Fermes de Marie

This minty warm infusion features coriander and aniseed—two surprising additions that give it a vaguely Mediterranean aroma. Feel free to reduce or leave out the stevia if you'd like—anise is a sweet spice that can make you think you're tasting sugar where there's none.

¼ bunch mint
10 whole coriander seeds
2 teaspoons aniseed
2 teaspoons stevia
  or raw honey
2 cups (240 ml) boiling
  filtered water
2 or 3 slices lemon

Put the mint, coriander, aniseed, and stevia in a teapot and add the boiling water. Let it infuse for about 10 minutes, then strain through a fine-mesh sieve and serve warm with lemon slices.

Makes one serving.

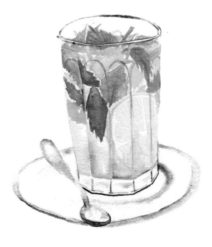

GREEN GRAPE ELIXIR

from Mathilde Thomas, founder, Caudalie

Exotic and unexpected flavors are all well and good, but sometimes
simplicity is best. Here, a minty fresh-pressed juice of grapes
and cucumber is simply topped off with sparkling water for a refreshing
thirst-quencher that's just barely sweet.

1 cup (150 g) green grapes
9 inches (23 cm) cucumber
1 sprig mint, stemmed, plus
  1 whole sprig for garnish
Cold sparkling water

Optional:
Ice cubes

Juice the grapes, cucumber, and mint leaves. Pour into
a tall glass, add ice cubes if you wish, and top off with
sparkling water. Garnish with a mint sprig and serve
immediately.

Makes one serving.

PASSION FRUIT GINGER HERBAL SODA

from Inge Theron, founder, Face Gym and the Spa Junkie

Did you know that the exotic fruit known as passion fruit contains 25 percent of your daily vitamin A needs plus pretty much all the vitamin C you need for a day, and is a great source of iron? Here it's blended up with some spicy ginger and sparkling water for an absolutely delicious, bubbly sweet treat. A splash of vodka would not be unwelcome here if the day calls for it.

3 passion fruits
2 inches (5 cm) fresh ginger
1 cup (240 ml) unsweetened coconut water
1 cup (240 ml) cold sparkling water
Mint leaves and fresh untreated rose petals for garnish

Optional:
Raw honey to taste

Juice the passion fruit and ginger. Stir in the coconut water and sparkling water. Serve immediately, poured over ice cubes or at room temperature with no ice, garnished with mint and rose petals. Stir in honey to taste, if desired.

Makes one serving.

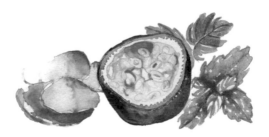

SPARKLING PIMM'S COCKTAIL
The Juicery

Flowery, tart, and fruity, this fabulous grown-up soda,
reminiscent of a Pimm's Cup, might become your go-to mocktail.

. . . .

½ cup (80 g) pitted cherries,
  plus more for garnish
¼ cup (40 g) blackberries,
  plus more for garnish
1 inch (2.5 cm) cucumber
1 slice lemon
5 to 6 mint leaves, plus more
  for garnish
1 cup (240 ml) sparkling
  water

Optional:
2 or 3 drops raw honey

Juice the cherries, blackberries, cucumber, lemon,
and mint. Top with the sparkling water. Stir in a few
drops honey, if using, and serve over ice and garnish
with cherries, blackberries, and mint.

Makes one serving.

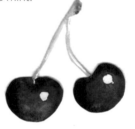

CUCUMBER BEET COCKTAIL
from Ananda in the Himalayas

Don't let the short ingredient list for this earthy, tart juice fool you.
Beets, cucumber, and lemon are three potent plant foods that can help
support liver function, improve circulation, and give your skin a boost.

. . . .

⅔ cup (180 g) beets
1 cup (80 g) cucumber
½ lemon, peeled
2 tablespoons cold sparkling
  water

Optional:
Ice cubes

Juice the beets, cucumber, and lemon. Stir in the
sparkling water. Serve immediately, over ice cubes if
you wish.

Makes one serving.

RED ENERGY JUICE
from Les Fermes de Marie

Red foods contain plenty of antioxidants. Raspberries are loaded with fiber, and strawberries are packed with vitamin C and folate. With a festive top-off of sparkling water, this tart drink is a healthful grown-up soda alternative.

1 small beet
½ cup (80 g) strawberries
½ cup (60 g) raspberries
A few mint leaves, plus
  1 for garnish
Cold sparkling water

Optional:
Ice cubes

Juice the beet. Transfer to a blender, add the strawberries, raspberries, and mint, and blend until smooth. Pour through a fine-mesh sieve into a tall glass, add ice if you wish, and top off with sparkling water. Garnish with a mint leaf and serve immediately.

Makes one serving.

CONTRIBUTORS

Christina Agnew
& Clare Neill
cofounders, Radiance
www.radiancecleanse.com

Ananda in the Himalayas
www.anandaspa.com

Cristiana Arcangeli
founder, Beauty'In
www.beautyin.com

Rick Bender
chef, Google NY/
Restaurant Associates
www.google.com
www.restaurantassociates.com

The Bloomsbury Hotel
www.doylecollection.com/
hotels/the-bloomsbury-hotel

Susan Blum, M.D.
director, Blum Center for
Health in Rye Brook, NY;
author, *The Immune System
Recovery Plan*
www.blumcenterforhealth.com

Brenners Park Hotel
and Spa
Baden Baden
www.brenners.com

Cal-a-Vie
www.cal-a-vie.com

Kris Carr, author,
and Chad Sarno, chef
Crazy Sexy Kitchen
www.kriscarr.com

Chiva-Som International
Health Resort
www.chivasom.com

Robert Ciborowski
executive chef, Westin Hotels
& Resorts, Walt Disney World
Swan and Dolphin Resort
www.westin.com

Kay Kay Clivio
instructor, Pure Yoga, New York
www.pureyoga.com

David A. Colbert, M.D.
founder and head physician,
New York Dermatology Group;
founder, Colbert MD Skincare
www.drdavidcolbert.com

Joe Cross
author, *Reboot with
Joe Juice Diet*; founder,
Reboot with Joe
www.fsnd.com
www.rebootwithjoe.com

Tiffany Cruikshank
Pure Yoga, New York
www.pureyoga.com

James Duigan
founder, Bodyism
www.bodyism.com

Julie Elliott
founder, In Fiore
www.infiore.net

Hala El-Shafie
founder, Nutrition Rocks
www.nutrition-rocks.co.uk

Les Fermes des Maries
www.fermesdemarie.com

Amelia Freer
nutritional therapist and founder,
Freer Nutrition
www.freernutrition.com

David Frenkiel
& Luise Vindahl
authors of *Green Kitchen
Stories* blog
www.greenkitchenstories.com

Melisse Gelula
& Alexia Brue
cofounders, Well+Good
www.wellandgoodnyc.com

Alex Glasscock
founder and owner,
The Ranch at Live Oak, Malibu
www.theranchmalibu.com

Schuyler Grant
cocreator, Wanderlust; director,
Kula Yoga Project
www.wanderlustfestival.com

Jason Harler
& Tanya Hughes
cofounders, American Medicinal
Arts, creators of holistic products
and spa experiences
www.americanmedicinalarts.com

Tata Harper
founder, Tata Harper Skincare
www.tataharperskincare.com

Jasmine &
Melissa Hemsley
founders, HEMSLEY +
HEMSLEY; authors,
The Art of Eating Well
www.hemsleyandhemsley.com

The Herb House
at Lime Wood
www.limewood.co.uk

Abigail James
international facialist and
well-being expert
www.abigailjames.com

Santosh Jori
executive chef, Westin
Hotels & Resorts, The Westin
Beijing Financial Street
www.westin.com

Dr. Alejandro Junger
medical director and creator,
The Clean Program
www.thecleanprogram.com

Dr. Naveen Kella
director and cofounder of
Urology & Prostate Institute,
Division of Oncology
San Antonio
www.texasroboticsurgery.com

The Kensington Hotel
www.doylecollection.com/
hotels/the-kensington-hotel

David Laris
founder, David Laris Creates
www.davidlariscreates.com

Dr. Frank Lipman
founder and director,
Eleven Eleven Wellness
Center and Be Well
www.drfranklipman.com
www.bewellbydrfranklipman.com

**Jennifer Maanavi
& Tanya Becker**
cofounders, Physique 57
www.physique57.com

The Marylebone Hotel
www.doylecollection.com/
hotels/the-marylebone-hotel

Moises Mehl
nood food Raw Food chef
www.allnood.com

Saimaa Miller
naturopath and author,
*Aussie Body Diet and Detox
Plan*, Aussie Body Diet Pty. Ltd.
www.thelastresort.com.au

Dr. Amy Myers
medical director and founder,
Amy Myers, M.D., Austin Ultra
Health
www.amymyersmd.com

Bobbi Neal
founder, The Joint Cafe,
and hospitality consultant
www.thejointcafe.com

Jess Ng
founder, ReOrient
www.drinkReOrient.com

Michelle Ngoh
cofounder, Yeotown
www.yeotown.com

Nini Ordoubadi
founder, Tay Tea
www.taytea.com

Cristina Paradelo
Shibui Spa at
The Greenwich Hotel
www.thegreenwichhotel.com

**Eve Persak, M.S., R.D.,
C.N.S.C., & Amanda Gale**
COMO Group executive chef
COMO Shambhala
www.comoshambhala.com

Marcelle Pick
R.N.C., M.S.N., OB/GYN
N.P., best-selling author and
cofounder, Women to Women
www.marcellepick.com

Alex Probyn
founder, Blends for Friends
www.blendsforfriends.com

Rosa Reisman
author and registered
nutritional consultant

Michelle Roques-O'Neil
aromatherapist, healer,
spiritual life coach, and
natural perfumer
www.roquesoneil.com

Kara Rosen
founder, Plenish Cleanse
www.plenishcleanse.com

Shonali Sabherwal
macrobiotic nutritionist,
chef, instructor, and founder,
Soulfood India
www.soulfoodshonali.com

Lior Lev Sercarz
chef, spice blender, and
founder, La Boîte
www.laboiteny.com

SHA Wellness Clinic
www.shawellnessclinic.com

Singita Spa
www.singita.com

Meghan Telpner
certified nutritional therapist
and director, Academy of
Culinary Nutrition

Inge Theron
founder, Face Gym and
the Spa Junkie
www.facegym.com

Mathilde Thomas
founder, Caudalie
www.caudalie.com

Vitamix
www.vitamix.com
Katrine van Wyk
author and holistic health
coach; nutrition consultant,
The Juicery
www.katrinevanwyk.com

Dalton Wong
founder, Twenty Two Training
www.twentytwotraining.com

Dr. Andrew Weil
True Kitchen
www.foxrc.com/restaurants/
true-food-kitchen/

Mark Zeitouni
executive chef,
Standard Hotel, Miami
www.standardhotels.com

RESOURCES

For the most up to date list of resources, please visit:

The Juicery
www.thejuiceryworld.com

JUICERS:

Breville
www.breville.com

Hurom
www.hurom.com

BLENDER:

Nutribullet
www.nutribullet.com

Vitamix
www.vitamix.com

FRENCH PRESS:

Bodum
www.bodum.com

PROTEIN POWDERS, SUPPLEMENTS & OTHER SPECIALTY ITEMS:

The Juicery
www.thejuiceryworld.com

Aduna
Baobab, the feel-good fruit from Africa! A naturally dried, nutrient-dense raw food used for centuries by Africans to promote well-being and beautiful skin.
www.aduna.com

BeWell by Dr. Frank Lipman
Healthy living made simple. Exceptional doctor-developed supplements and cleanse program that is both easy to follow and incredibly effective. Supplements, detox support, shakes, and coaching.
www.bewellbydrfranklipman.com

Bodyism Clean and Lean Supplements
Bodyism specializes in creating long, lean, athletic bodies by building health through customized nutritional protocols and movement and exercise programs along with a bespoke range of supplements.
www.bodyism.com

The Chia Co.
Pure and nutrient-dense superfoods. The Chia Co. grows its seeds on sustainable, chemical-free farms in western Australia.
www.thechiaco.co.au

The Clean Program
A twenty-one-day detox, cleanse, and diet designed by Dr. Alejandro Junger. It is the most endorsed, supported, and effective cleanse in the world.
www.thecleanprogram.com

Jax Coco
Premium, all-natural coconut products, sustainably sourced. Including 100 percent pure microfiltered coconut water, never from concentrate, in an elegant glass bottle.
www.jaxcoco.com

Tay Tea
Exclusive, hand-blended artisanal tea, founded by tea blender Nini Ordoubadi— 100 percent natural and wild crafted.
www.taytea.com

Naturya
The most popular nutrient-rich, antioxidant-packed power foods from around the world. Additive-free, single-ingredient products. Vegan and organic.
www.naturya.com

Navitas Naturals - The Superfood Company
The mission of Navitas Naturals is to provide the finest organic superfoods that increase energy and enhance health. Since 2003, health-conscious people have been choosing these organic superfoods because they're a diverse whole-food source of antioxidants, protein, essential fats, minerals, vitamins and other key nutrients.
www.navitasnaturals.com

Organic Burst
Organic superfood supplements.
www.organicburst.com

INDEX